Cracking the General Surgical Interviews for ST3

Cracking the General Surgical Interviews for ST3

Sala Abdalla BSc MBBS FRCS (Gen Surg)
Consultant General and Upper Gastrointestinal Surgeon
London North West University Healthcare Trust

Amber Shivarajan BMedSci BMBS MRCS
Specialty Training Registrar—ST3
South East London General Surgery Training Programme

Kaushiki Singh BSc MBBS MRCS
Specialty Training Registrar—ST4
South East London General Surgery Training Programme

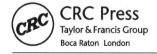

CRC Press
Taylor & Francis Group
Boca Raton London

CRC Press is an imprint of the
Taylor & Francis Group, an **informa** business

First edition published 2022
by CRC Press
6000 Broken Sound Parkway NW, Suite 300, Boca Raton, FL 33487–2742

and by CRC Press
2 Park Square, Milton Park, Abingdon, Oxon, OX14 4RN

© 2022 Taylor & Francis Group, LLC

CRC Press is an imprint of Taylor & Francis Group, LLC

Library of Congress Cataloging-in-Publication Data
Names: Abdalla, Sala, author. | Shivarajan, Amber, author. | Singh, Kaushiki, author.
Title: Cracking the general surgical interviews for ST3 / Sala Abdalla, Amber Shivarajan, Kaushiki Singh.
Description: First edition. | Boca Raton : CRC Press, 2022. | Includes bibliographical references and index.
Identifiers: LCCN 2021040178 (print) | LCCN 2021040179 (ebook) | ISBN 9781032073262 (paperback) |
    ISBN 9781032118352 (hardback) | ISBN 9781003221739 (ebook)
Subjects: MESH: General Surgery—education | Education, Medical, Graduate | Interviews as Topic—methods |
    United Kingdom
Classification: LCC RD27.85 (print) | LCC RD27.85 (ebook) | NLM WO 18 | DDC 617.0071—dc23
LC record available at https://lccn.loc.gov/2021040178
LC ebook record available at https://lccn.loc.gov/2021040179

ISBN: 978-1-032-11835-2 (hbk)
ISBN: 978-1-032-07326-2 (pbk)
ISBN: 978-1-003-22173-9 (ebk)

DOI: 10.1201/9781003221739

Typeset in Times
by Apex CoVantage, LLC

Contents

Contents

Foreword

Preparation for interview for specialty training in general surgery can be quite daunting. There is a paucity of information on how best to approach this important event, and there are no formal guidelines on how best to prepare.

Cracking the general surgical interviews for ST3 is unique, for it provides a comprehensive framework for future trainees to work with. This book is elegantly written by three young surgeons at different spectra of their surgical careers, hence covering all aspects of the interview process and offering an insight into the interviewers' perspective. The interview process has changed over the years, and having three surgeons at different stages of their careers provides a wholesome perspective of what is expected of the potential candidate.

The authors have diligently addressed every aspect of the ST3 interview process in a logical manner and offered practical advice at each station. The section on the portfolio station provides a platform for future candidates to model their curriculum vitaes on. The clinical sections are exemplary and cover a wide breadth of surgical conditions with an in-depth mini revision quality. Additionally, the authors have provided an outline of the mandatory courses that the candidates need to have attended and how the learning points from those courses can be integrated into clinical practice. There is an exhaustive section on ethics and how to manage the patient with learning difficulties; questions on safeguarding are a common pitfall for candidates. The final section on preparation for the interview during the COVID era is in keeping with present times.

This book is an instructive read for future candidates, especially overseas graduates who are not familiar with the system. It helps allay the element of fear of the unknown and enables the candidate to approach the interview with confidence. This excellent book will be a good read for those who conduct the interviews too as it offers structure and an idea of the applicants' perspective of the interview process.

Through this book, the authors have equipped future applicants for ST3 in general and vascular surgery with the knowledge, structure and confidence that are needed to succeed in their quest.

Tayo Oke MMedSci, FRCS (Gen Surg), FRCS (Ed)
Consultant Colorectal Surgeon
Queen Elizabeth Hospital, London

Preface

ST3 interviews are national interviews that all doctors wishing to enroll in higher surgical training (ST3–ST8 stages) in the United Kingdom are required to take. If they succeed in these structured interviews, they are awarded a national training number. ST3 interviews are extremely competitive, and achieving the highest possible score is essential in securing the post of your choice. In 2020 there were 574 applicants for 123 posts in general and vascular surgery nationally.

The key to success in these interviews is diligent preparation. Indeed, the lead author's belief is that these interviews should be prepared for like an exam. While preparing for her own ST3 interviews some years ago, she found that there was very little published material to guide her. Even today, most of the available textbooks are generic to all medical disciplines with minimal focus on general surgery. Candidates for the most part resort to using multiple sources for their preparation. This book started off as her own set of notes which she has formulated into a comprehensive textbook directed towards the general surgical ST3 interviews.

This book outlines the structure and format of the current ST3 general surgical interviews, with chapters dedicated to each area that is assessed on the day. There is a detailed focus on the portfolio station, drawing in from the first-hand experience of the authors. In the chapters on clinical and clinical management, the emphasis is placed not only on the clinical content but also on the organization of thoughts and delivery of answers. Through numerous clinical examples, the candidate is equipped with a framework for tackling any clinical question they may encounter beyond the scope of this book. At the end of each clinical and clinical management scenario, a list of topics is outlined for suggested further reading. There are additional chapters on technical skills scenarios, principles of research and audit and medical ethics which have featured in previous ST3 interviews. The final chapter outlines tips on interview technique and helpful pointers from the authors and past candidates which are applicable to both face-to-face and online interviews.

Written in an engaging style, this book provides essential guidance for the reader with all the required material in one single textbook, a bonus for many candidates who have little time to comb through various sources with their demanding work schedules. It is aimed at instilling the readers with the tools and confidence needed to succeed at the ST3 general surgical and vascular interview.

About the Authors

Sala Abdalla BSc MBBS FRCS (Gen Surg)
Sala Abdalla is a London-based Consultant General and Upper Gastrointestinal Surgeon. She graduated from Imperial College, London, and completed her higher surgical training in South East London. She is very active in medical education and her contributions include the redeveloping of the Royal College of Surgeons of England's Intermediate Laparoscopic Skills course and training junior surgeons on the Core Skills in Laparoscopy and Basic Surgical Skills courses. She has a special interest in humanitarian work and has led surgical missions to low- and middle-income countries. Sala Abdalla is the coauthor of "A History of Surgery" with Harold Ellis, emeritus professor of surgery. This book began as her set of notes while preparing for a national training number in general surgery. There was, and still is, a paucity of books focused on these highly competitive interviews. She hopes that the readers will now have a comprehensive resource in supporting them to succeed in their ST3 interviews.

Amber Shivarajan BMedSci BMBS MRCS
Amber Shivarajan graduated from the University of Nottingham with an intercalated Bachelor of Science degree in 2014 and a degree in Bachelor of Medicine and Surgery in 2016. She completed her post-graduate foundation and junior surgical training in hospitals around Greater Manchester and South London. She has worked as a Junior Clinical Research Fellow in Upper GI, HPB and Bariatric Surgery at King's College Hospital, London. While preparing for the ST3 interviews in general surgery, she found Sala Abdalla's notes very informative and suggested they be adapted into a book. Using these notes, she was able to secure a national training number in general surgery in London as well as her first-choice rotation.

Kaushiki Singh BSc MBBS MRCS
Kaushiki Singh has a medical degree from King's College, London, and an intercalated Bachelor of Science degree in medical management from Imperial College, London. She completed her foundation training in London and core surgical training in Portsmouth. She excelled at the ST3 interviews and went on to receive her first-choice rotation. She is currently working as ST4 Registrar in general surgery in South East London. She cites the breadth of knowledge as one of the challenges in preparing for ST3 interviews and hopes that this book will be the all-in-one resource to helping candidates prepare and succeed.

Acknowledgments

This book is dedicated to Sam for her unwavering support over countless years. I am also grateful to my two contributors who have worked tirelessly amidst hectic work schedules to shape this book. They are to be congratulated for their valuable contribution. A final word of gratitude to my good friend and champion, Professor Harold Ellis CBE FRCS.

Sala Abdalla

I would like to dedicate this book to my good friends Julia and James, for their immeasurable support and positivity during this challenging year. I also wish to extend my gratitude to my coauthor, friend and mentor, Sala, without whom none of this would have been possible.

Amber Shivarajan

I am grateful to Bandana and Uday for their faith in me. It has also been a pleasure to share this experience with Amber and Sala.

Kaushiki Singh

Format of the Interview

Traditionally, the interview for entry into higher surgical training consisted of stations to assess the domains covered in the general surgical ST3 person specification. These stations were grouped into portfolio, professional communication, clinical, clinical management, technical skills, leadership and teamwork, and academic. In 2020, due to the COVID-19 pandemic, this process was modified to reflect the national safety precaution measures, and selection for ST3 was based purely on the candidates' self-assessment of their portfolio. In 2021, with the widespread uptake of telemedicine, the selection process was expanded to include a virtual interview. This consisted of a clinical, clinical management, and portfolio stations, each lasting ten minutes. A five-minute preparation station was given for candidates to read each of the clinical and clinical management scenarios. Regardless of the format, the assessment criteria have largely remained similar over the last ten years. As such, changes to the structure should not hamper your preparation.

PREPARING FOR THE INTERVIEW

Interview preparation should allow you to build, enhance and consolidate the knowledge and skills amassed during your core training or equivalent years. To prepare well, it is essential to understand what qualities you are expected to demonstrate.

A good starting point is reading and understanding the person specification. This document can be found on the oriel website and outlines specific qualities required for progression to ST3 (https://specialtytraining.hee.nhs.uk/Recruitment/Person-specifications).

After reviewing this document, you will need to consider the role of the examiner. This can be broken down into the following criteria:

- To assess the candidate's clinical judgment and ability to handle challenging clinical management scenarios
- To check that the candidate matches their portfolio
- To allow the candidate to enhance aspects of their portfolio and gain extra marks
- To assess the candidate's understanding of the broader role as a surgeon (leadership, research, ethics)
- To ascertain if the candidate is a safe surgeon

Finally, you must have a good understanding of the content of each station. Next is a brief introduction to each of the stations, and this will be followed by dedicated chapters outlining each station's content and preparation in detail.

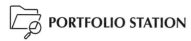 PORTFOLIO STATION

The portfolio station aims to assess your ability to meet the person specifications. You will have 15 minutes of questions on the following topics:

- Achievements and experience in each domain
- Commitment to surgery
- Desired career progression
- A little bit about yourself

Traditionally, the candidate's portfolio is reviewed by the panelist for 5 minutes before the interview. For the 2021 entry, the portfolio was not provided to the interviewer. However, as interviews were recorded, any questions regarding the candidate's probity could be verified later. You must ensure all information provided is accurate and not misleading.

 Tips:

- Organize and prepare your curriculum vitae and portfolio in advance using the person specification
- Be concise and consolidate the evidence (feedback, comments)
- Ensure the portfolio is clearly laid out and easy to navigate
- Know your portfolio inside out
- Have specific examples for each domain, commitment to specialty and what you are most proud of

Refer to Chapter 1 for more detailed information on how to prepare for this station.

 # CLINICAL STATION

This station comprises clinical scenarios which involve the assessment and management of surgical patients in different clinical settings. Preparation for this station requires a systematic approach that will be outlined further in Chapter 2.

 # CLINICAL MANAGEMENT STATION

In the clinical management station, the emphasis is on your ability to use your management skills to solve clinical problems. It aims to assess whether you can think beyond the clinical dilemma to other aspects of care such as prioritization and availability of resources. The marking scheme is similar to that in the clinical station. Further details are available in Chapter 3.

The following table outlines the marking scheme for this station:

Criteria	Scoring
Recognition of the clinical issues	1—Poor
Judgment and prioritization	2—Area for concern
Planning and use of investigations and/or resources	3—Satisfactory
Communication strategy	4—Good
	5—Excellent

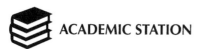

ACADEMIC STATION

This station assesses your understanding of research, research principles and your ability to critically appraise a research article. You will be provided with an abstract or research article and given time to read and prepare. You will be expected to provide a summary, review the article's positive and negative aspects, and then you'll be asked questions related to it. You may also be asked to define the audit cycle and related terms.

 Tips:

- Develop a structure for presenting your appraisal of the article or abstract
- Practice preparing summaries for abstracts and research articles
- Learn about the different study designs, common statistical terms and guidelines such as PRISMA, CONSORT and STROBE
- Review the definition of clinical governance and other related definitions such as "audit" and the "audit cycle"

Chapter 4 has more details on how to prepare for this station.

TECHNICAL SKILLS STATION

Candidates will be asked to demonstrate a surgical skill. This will most likely be an example of what is encountered in the Royal College of Surgeons Basic Surgical Skills or Core Skills in Laparoscopic surgery course. You may be required to teach the surgical skill to the examiner as if they were a junior doctor or a medical student. Refer to Chapter 5 for more detailed information on how to prepare for this station.

ETHICS STATION

Although there is no formal ethics station, ethical dilemmas can be presented in clinical and clinical management scenarios. In some situations, the ethical dilemma may not be apparent, and you will have to dissect the scenario carefully to identify these issues. Certain ethical concepts such as consent and capacity are highly relevant to day-to-day surgical practice, and therefore it is worth spending time reviewing these. Chapter 6 covers ethics in great detail.

Finally, and once again, preparation for the interview is the key to your success. Each of the detailed chapters in this book is designed to help you prepare, but there is no substitute for hard graft. This is your best opportunity to make a good impression on the interviewers and show them what you have to offer. Enjoy it, and best of luck!

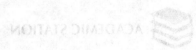

ACADEMIC STATION

This station assesses your understanding of research, research principles, and your ability to critically appraise a research article. You will be provided with an abstract or research article and given time to read and interpret. You will be expected to provide a summary, review the article's positive and negative aspects, and then will be asked questions about the research. You may also be asked to define the null hypothesis and related terms.

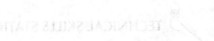

Tips

- Develop a structure for presenting your appraisal of the article or abstract.
- Practice preparing summaries for abstracts and research articles.
- Learn about the different study designs, common statistical terms and guidelines such as PRISMA, CONSORT and STROBE.
- Review the definition of clinical governance, and other related definitions such as "audit" and the "audit cycle".

Chapter 8 has more details on how to prepare for this station.

TECHNICAL SKILLS STATION

Candidates will be asked to demonstrate a surgical skill. This will most likely be an example of what is encountered in the Royal College of Surgeons Basic Surgical Skills or Core Skills in Laparoscopic Surgery course. You may be asked to use this surgical skill in the examination or there were a number of more complex skills. Refer to Chapter 5 for more detailed information on how to prepare for this station.

ETHICS STATION

Medicine throughout must adhere to ethical and legal frameworks to be practised in a legal and clinical management scenarios. In some situations, the ethical dilemmas may not be unusual, and you will have to dissect the pros and legality to identify these issues. Certain ethical complications are common and commonly are highly relevant to day-to-day surgical practice, and therefore it is worth spending time reviewing these. Chapter 6 covers ethics in great detail.

Finally, and once again, preparation for the interview is the key to your success. Each of the detailed chapters in this book is designed to help you prepare, but there is no substitute for hard graft. This is your best opportunity to make a good impression on the interviewers and show them what you have to offer. Think of it as your best moment.

1 Portfolio Station

The portfolio is one of the critical components of the ST3 recruitment process. It is a collection of evidence designed to show that the applicant meets the person specification requirements for the specialist training program in general and vascular surgery.

 THE PERSON SPECIFICATION

The person specification for ST3 sets out the desirable traits and achievements that the ideal candidate would have. It is released every year and is worth reading to help you prepare for the interview. Here is a summary of the key points in the person specification.

The ideal candidate would demonstrate evidence of the following:

- **Career progression**

  - Achievement of the competencies as listed in the Core Surgical Training Curriculum

- **Clinical skills**

  - Application of sound clinical knowledge and judgment to problems
  - Appropriate prioritization of clinical need
  - Technical and clinical competence
  - Diagnostic skills and clinical judgment

- **Research and audit skills**
  - Understanding of audit, clinical risk management and evidence-based practice
  - Knowledge of basic research principles, methodology and ethics
  - Contribution to audit

- **Teaching**

  - Participation in teaching others

- **Communication skills**

  - Ability to communicate with others productively and considerately
  - Ability to discuss management options with patients in an effective manner

- **Problem-solving and decision-making**

  - The use of a range of problem-solving methods
  - Development of suitable judgment and decision-making skills

DOI: 10.1201/9781003221739-1

- **Managing others and team involvement**
  - Leadership skills
  - Management skills
  - Working successfully with colleagues and in a multidisciplinary team

- **Organizing and planning**
  - Time management and appropriate prioritization of workload
  - Ability to balance urgent demands and follow instructions
  - Understanding the importance and use of information systems

- **Vigilance and situational awareness**
  - Anticipating situations that may arise and preparing for them accordingly

- **Coping with pressure and managing uncertainty**
  - Working efficiently under pressure
  - Working effectively in highly emotive situations
  - Being aware of one's limitations
  - Knowing when to ask for help

- **Values**
  - Knowledge of the values of the national health service (NHS) which are:
    - Improving lives
    - Commitment to quality of care
    - Respect and dignity
    - Compassion
    - Working together for patients

- **Probity**
  - Taking responsibility for their actions
  - Understanding ethical principles including safety, confidentiality and consent

- **Commitment to specialty**
  - Having a realistic insight into general and vascular surgery and the personal demands of training in surgery
  - Understanding the training program
  - Being committed to one's development

The various aspects of the portfolio and the questions that can be asked in the portfolio station are designed to elicit the various features listed in the specification.

 THE PORTFOLIO

The portfolio is fully prepared and submitted before the interview, and so it is the one part of the interview process which can be controlled entirely by the applicant. Early preparation is vital for success in the portfolio station. The portfolio requirements are updated each year and can be found in the applicant's handbook on the specialty recruitment website. It is essential to read this handbook before the application to ensure that the current standards are met.

Overall, there are specific portfolio requirements that do not change significantly from year to year. This chapter will cover the separate areas of the portfolio in detail. The portfolio station requirements for several previous years have been analyzed, and details have been provided on each requirement. The portfolio station for any given year will include a combination of these.

It is necessary to start preparing evidence for the portfolio at least several months, ideally years, in advance. Evidence can be used from the beginning of medical training.

Awareness of the requirements of the portfolio is essential so that any missing areas can be acquired before the interview.

THE FORMAT OF THE PORTFOLIO STATION

There are two aspects to the portfolio station. The first is the content of the portfolio which will be assessed and marked. Usually, the portfolio is submitted ahead of the interview. The second aspect is your ability to answer questions about your career in general. The candidate will usually spend 10 minutes answering such questions.

The first part of this chapter looks at the portfolio requirements, and the second part looks at the questions that may be asked.

Portfolio requirements and evidence which can be supplied for each

1. 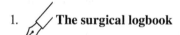 **The surgical logbook**

   - This section is an important part and looks at the numbers of index procedures performed by the applicant.
   - These numbers should be recorded in an electronic format. A consolidation sheet from a validated logbook can be used as evidence of the number of procedures performed by the applicant. Electronic 'E'-logbook is an example of a standard website used for this purpose in the United Kingdom.
   - The 'index procedures' are the essential procedures that applicants to the specialty training program are expected to have. These procedures can vary from year to year and include appendicectomies (laparoscopic and/or open), repair of inguinal hernias, emergency laparotomy, groin exploration, laparotomy incision and closure, laparoscopic port placement and closure, and cholecystectomy. Appendicectomies and inguinal hernias make the list each year, so these are the two procedures to mainly target during clinical placements before the interview.
   - Different points can be given to the number of these procedures performed and whether they were performed supervised or unsupervised by the trainer.

- Work-based assessments (WBAs) such as DOPS (direct observation of procedural skills) or PBAs (procedure-based assessments) signed off by consultants can be used to supplement the logbook evidence—these are forms available on the intercollegiate surgical curriculum programme (ISCP) website. Often, a higher number of points are available for WBAs performed at a level 3 or 4 which denote greater competence. This section aims to show the acquisition of at least a CT2 level skill in these procedures.

2. Publications

- Only papers that have been published in PubMed-indexed journals and have a PMID (PubMed identifier) are awarded points.
- These can include papers published during medical school or previous degrees.
- Case reports receive fewer points, and in some years, they have not been included at all in the assessment.
- Published abstracts, letters or technical tips are not included here.
- Maximum points are available for first author publications, although some points may still be awarded for authorship in any other position on the author list.

3. Presentations

- These include oral or poster presentations given at regional, national, or international conferences.
- The candidate must be a listed author for the presentation to be eligible for points.
- It is worthwhile submitting presentations each year to conferences such as ASIT (Association of Surgeons in Training) annual conference and the ASGBI (Association of Surgeons of Great Britain and Ireland) annual conference which highly encourage trainee input.
- Maximum points are available for oral national and international presentations.
- In some years, only oral presentations have scored points, so this is a good area to focus effort on.

4. Audits

- This section is an excellent opportunity to maximize points as audits can easily be performed during clinical placements.
- Maximum points are available for closed-loop audit cycles.

- It is worthwhile performing as many audits as possible and closing the cycle prior to the interview to gain maximum points.
- Active involvement in the audit process will need to be demonstrated.
- Each Trust has an audit department with which the audit needs to be registered. This department can usually provide evidence of audit activity in the form of a certificate.
- Examples of audits that can be completed during clinical placements include appropriate completion of consent forms for patients, proper prescribing of antibiotics for patients, and documentation of the NELA (National Emergency Laparotomy Audit) predicted mortality rate before an emergency laparotomy.

5. Further degrees

- This includes degrees that have been awarded by the time of application.
- Maximum points are usually granted for a completed PhD or MD with slightly fewer points available for a Master's or a Bachelor's degree.
- The fewest points are typically awarded to intercalated or incomplete degrees.

6. Leadership

- This can be within medicine or outside of medicine.
- Evidence of a formal leadership or management role will need to be provided.
- Examples of leadership include a certificate for being the rota manager for your department, a certificate for organizing your department's weekly teaching/grand rounds or monthly morbidity and mortality meeting, roles as local/regional/national trainee representative, committee member of a local/regional/national medical society and involvement in organizing regional meetings such as an audit evening for your deanery.
- Points are also available for courses undertaken on leadership.

7. Teaching

- Maximum points are available for a formal qualification in teaching, such as a postgraduate certificate.
- Points are also available for teaching-based courses such as attendance at the Training the Trainer course
- Points are also awarded for provision of regular formal teaching such as weekly departmental teaching or medical student teaching.

- Evidence for involvement in teaching will need to be provided, e.g. a certificate from the head of the department to show involvement in regular teaching.

8. **Courses**

- The courses usually required for completion of Core Surgical Training are Advanced Trauma Life Support (ATLS), Basic Surgical Skills (BSS) and Care of the Critically Ill Surgical Patient (CCrISP) courses.
- In addition to these, points are sometimes available for completing extra courses relevant to the specialty e.g. Core Skills in Laparoscopic surgery course.
- A maximum of six extra courses in addition to ATLS, BSS and CCrISP are usually considered excluding leadership or management courses (these are awarded points elsewhere).

9. **Awards/prizes**

- These can include an undergraduate prize or primary medical degree with honours.
- Local or regional postgraduate prizes are also considered, so it is worthwhile applying for competitions that trusts or local/regional surgical societies run.
- Maximum points are available for national and international prizes e.g. Royal College of Surgeon's exam prize, the Annual Professor Harold Ellis Medical Student Prize for Surgery and Moynihan Prize.

ADJUSTMENTS TO POINTS

An adjustment is usually made to the scores to reflect the number of years of experience an applicant has relative to their achievements. For example if an applicant has less than four years of experience since their medical degree, their base score will multiply by a higher number than an applicant who has more years of experience. This is to make the process more equitable when comparing candidates with different years of experience and training backgrounds.

PORTFOLIO PRESENTATION

Traditionally, the portfolio was required as a hard copy on the day of the interview. In recent years, evidence for the portfolio has been uploaded online. Regardless of the method chosen, there are specific key points to adhere to when preparing the portfolio:

- Have the evidence present in a typed format

- Have the applicant's name and GMC number present at the bottom of each page
- Have a clear and concise contents page at the beginning
- Have dividers that specify each section of the portfolio
- Have page numbers present on each page which correspond to the contents page at the beginning
- Points are only gained in the portfolio if the interviewers can find the relevant piece of evidence, therefore the evidence has to be presented clearly
- Ensure correct spellings and appropriate grammar throughout

CHANGES DUE TO THE COVID-19 PANDEMIC

Throughout the Covid-19 pandemic, the portfolio was a key feature of the interview process and has been largely based on self-assessment. The mark sheet was provided online, and the applicant had to go through the sections and allocate themselves points based on their evidence. In the 2020 application process, a certain percentage of applicants had their evidence formally re-checked. In the 2021 interviews, all applicants had their evidence checked, and those who achieved beyond a certain mark were invited to a virtual interview by the panel.

There will always be a portfolio station within the interview in some format or other. Self-assessment for the portfolio is highly likely to be just a short-term adjustment for the pandemic. The core content of what the portfolio station requires will not change drastically over time.

A NOTE ON PROBITY

Falsifying information in the portfolio is a serious offense and will lead to the applicant being reported to the General Medical Council. The applicant must ensure that all the evidence submitted can be confirmed. Any patient-identifiable information must be omitted (name, address).

THE MARK SHEET

Tabel 1 shows an example mark sheet that is based on the 2019 interview. It gives an overview of how the portfolio may be scored. The sections included and the points awarded may differ slightly each year. The applicant is advised to refer to the most recent mark sheet available that is likely to feature in their interview.

 PORTFOLIO STATION—EXAMPLE QUESTIONS

In this part of the interview, the interviewers have 10 minutes to ask about the applicant's career to date and seek to determine whether the applicant possesses the desirable traits.

There are specific frameworks that can be used to help answer questions in this station. It is important to practice using these frameworks before the interview.

TABLE 1

Requirements	Score 1	Score 2	Score 3	Score 4	Score 5
Postgraduate degrees	Degree in progress, i.e. one module completed	BSc or BA awarded MD/MS/PhD in progress (1 year completed)	MD/MS/PhD in progress (2 years completed)	Master's degree awarded MD/MD/PhD submitted	MD/MS/PhD awarded
Academic prizes	MBBS with Honours 1 undergraduate prize	>1 undergraduate prize	1 postgraduate prize	>1 postgraduate prize	International prize
Evidence of clinical experience (WBAs)	CT1 level, i.e. MSF, mini-CEX or CBDs demonstrating this	CT2 level WBAs	Some WBAs above CT2 level	At least 5 WBAs at level 3	At least 5 WBAs at level 4 with multiple consultant ratings
Evidence of technical experience (logbook and PBAs)	Logbook at CT1 level—assisting	Some cases at CT2 level	All cases at CT2 level	At least 5 index procedures at level 3 or 4	Multiple index procedures at level 4
Courses (in general or vascular surgery)	2 of ATLS, BSS or CCrISP completed and 1 extra course for each year beyond Core Training	ATLS, BSS and CCrISP and 1 extra course for each year beyond Core Training	ATLS, BSS, CCrISP and 2 extra courses	ATLS, BSS, CCrISP and 4 extra courses	ATLS, BSS, CCrISP and 6 extra courses
Audit (each requires personal involvement)	2 audits without a completed cycle	2 audits and one full cycle completed	3 audits with 2 cycles completed or 4 audits with one full cycle or 5 audits without cycle completion	5 audits with 3 full cycles or 6 audits with 2 full cycles or 8 audits without cycle completion	>6 audits with 4 full cycles or 10 audits without cycle completion
Publications	2 case reports or 1 publication as a coauthor	1 significant author peer-reviewed paper or >2 publications as a coauthor	>2 significant author publications	>4 significant author publications	>7 significant author publications
Presentations	1 regional oral or poster presentation	1 national/international oral or 3 poster	2 national/international oral or 6 poster or 1 oral and 3 poster	5 national/international oral	>7 national/international oral
Teaching	Ward-based teaching	Regular ward-based teaching or 1-day course completed	2-day course completed or Single lecture or regular tutorials (at least 2 needed)	>3 lectures with feedback or ATLS instructor or involvement in curriculum development	Lecture series delivered or leading role in a course/curriculum development
Management and leadership	Organizing rotas or day leadership course or student Rep role	Regular local meeting organizer, i.e. MDTs	Local trainee Rep Committee member of a local medical society	Organized regional meetings or regional Rep or committee member of a national medical society	National Rep role or president of a national medical society

ANSWERING QUESTIONS ABOUT YOUR BACKGROUND AND MOTIVATION

Examples of such questions are:

- Tell me about yourself
- Why do you want to train in general or vascular surgery?
- What are you particularly proud of in your portfolio?
- Where do you see yourself in 5 or 10 years?

The **CAMP** framework can be used for answering these types of questions:

C—Clinical = work experience, clinical interests, clinical skills
A—Academic = research, teaching experience, further education
M—Management = leadership/management experience
P—Personal = interests, extra-curricular activities

Example

Tell me about yourself?

I am a CT2 level Doctor currently working in general surgery. I have a year's experience in general surgery jobs at several district general hospitals. I have also worked in urology and plastic surgery. I am passionate about general surgery and have tried to gain as much experience as possible in this specialty. I have performed ten appendicectomies at a PBA (procedural-based assessment) level 3 standard, and have assisted with 20 laparotomies. I am also keen to do research and have published a literature review as first author on the management of seromas in breast surgery. I am currently working towards a Master's degree in laparoscopic surgery. Outside of medicine, I am a keen badminton player and organize my local badminton club matches.

The applicant should know the contents of their portfolio in detail and provide a summary if asked. Answers should be prepared for each section of the can be answered:

- What is your teaching experience?
- What is your management/leadership experience?
- What is your operative experience?
- What is your research/audit experience?

COMPETENCY-BASED QUESTIONS

Examples of these include the following:

- Tell me about your experiences in the following: working in a team/working under pressure/using your management skills
- What are your strengths/weaknesses?
- What would you say has been your best achievement to date?
- How do you handle stress?

The **STAR** framework can be used to formulate examples for these questions asked about particular traits:

S—Situation = What is the background to the story?
T—Task = What did you have to achieve?
A—Action = What did you do? How and why?
R—Result = What was the end outcome? Reflect on this.

Spend time talking about the action and the result, as this is where the appropriate personality traits are demonstrated for the interviewer's benefit.

Example:

Give us an example of when you've demonstrated leadership

> *I volunteered during the London 2012 Olympic Games during the field hockey tournament. I had to ensure that the temporary seating stands did not get overcrowded as there would be a risk of people falling over. I delegated specific tasks to my team and then regularly went back and checked that the tasks had been performed adequately. I also ensured that my team members understood and felt competent with the jobs they had been asked to perform. We finished the event with no incidents. I learnt how to adapt my leadership style to the problem at hand.*

Hot Topics and Themes

The following are common topics and themes that candidates need to be familiar with before the interview

 AUDIT

- **What is your definition of an audit?**
  An audit is a process that compares clinical practice against the current gold standard. The purpose of an audit is to enable clinicians to constantly improve their practice and therefore provide the best level of care for their patients.
- **What is an audit cycle, and what does this entail?**

  An audit cycle is a process that sees an audit being completed where changes have been implemented and re-audited. It consists of the following steps:

  1. Select the area for improvement.

     This can be any area in clinical practice where problems have arisen, i.e. identified through complaints, the occurrence of mistakes, staff concerns, etc.

  2. Identify the gold standard criteria/guidelines.

     Draw standards from the best available evidence, such as evidence set by NICE (National Institute for Health and Clinical Excellence), the relevant Royal Colleges, and the relevant Trusts. The idea is to check compliance with the standards.

3. Collect data on current practice.

Collect data within a pre-agreed timeframe for a specific group of individuals (anonymized). Data can be collected with the aid of the Trust's clinical audit department (can collect notes, help with statistical analysis and help with the presentation of data). All audits must be registered with the Trust's audit department.

4. Compare this data to the standards to determine how well the criteria have been met.

If standards have not been met, then the reasons for this should be identified as this will provide the potential for improving clinical practice.

5. Implement the appropriate changes.

This is the step that aims to improve the practice. Changes will need to be made, such as altering protocols, altering roles/responsibilities and improving documentation.

6. Close the loop—re-audit (completing the audit cycle).

Once the changes have been implemented, and after an agreed period has passed, so the changes have had time to impact, clinical practice should be audited again to measure the impact of the changes. A re-audit should use the same methods and data analysis. The re-audit should show that the standards have been matched. If not, further changes and further re-audits will need to be implemented.

- **What are the advantages of the audit process?**
  - The audit process enables the standard of care in a department or hospital to be improved and matched to the agreed gold standard. It helps staff identify pitfalls within their work processes and develop suitable solutions for them. This leads to a continuous cycle of improvement.
  - Audit data can also provide information to the hospital, the board of governors, patients and the Department of Health about the quality of care provided by a service. This also enables the development of other departments/hospitals. An audit is also a good training tool for junior doctors to learn about quality improvement principles.

- **What are the disadvantages of the audit process?**
  - At a departmental level, the audit will identify changes that are required, but other team members may resist these changes. The changes may also require complex and time-consuming solutions. It can also be challenging to acquire the relevant data.
  - At a trust level, the audits performed by junior doctors may not be against the standards that the Trust wishes to audit. Also, as junior doctors change jobs every 4–6 months, there will be a loss of continuity in the audit, so the cycle may not be completed.

- At a national level, the results from one Trust may not apply to other trusts as each Trust tends to have its specific guidelines, procedures and challenges.

- **What would you say is the difference between audit and research?**

  - Audit compares clinical practice against current standards of care while research aims to develop new standards of care by creating knowledge. An audit is practice-driven and continuous, whereas research is a one-off process. Research may involve experimentation, whereas audits are data-gathering exercises. Research usually requires ethical approval, while audits rarely do. Research is based on a hypothesis while an audit measures the extent to which the best standards are adhered to.

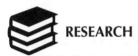 **RESEARCH**

- **Why is research necessary?**

  - It drives medical advancement and creates a pool of knowledge that can be translated into better patient care. Patients benefit directly through improved treatments.
  - A Trust involved in trials can provide patients with early access to the latest technology, enhancing the Trust's reputation.
  - A junior doctor involved in research gains education on the evidence on which decisions are made, e.g. treatments and procedures. It allows for continual professional development by keeping them up to date with current published research. It enables them to gain numerous skills such as organizational skills, writing and presentation skills.

- **What are the drawbacks of research?**

  - Much research does not get published, and many research projects do not get completed due to a lack of time or lack of funding.
  - Taking time out of clinical practice to do research poses the risk of deskilling, particularly if the research period is extended.

- **What is research governance?**

  Research governance is the framework whereby a set of standards of good practice and regulations are applied to research.

  Key features include:

  - Approval of research by an ethics committee
  - Informed consent from patients or subjects participating in the research
  - Patient dignity and safety is paramount
  - Confidentiality toward patient data
  - Review of the current evidence
  - Research proposals must be peer-reviewed

- Information about research must be carried out
- Organization of finance

 ## CLINICAL GOVERNANCE

- **What is clinical governance?**

  - It is a process that sets out principles for clinicians to follow to achieve the best level of care for their patients and ensure continuous quality improvement.

- **What are the seven pillars of clinical governance?**

A good pneumonic for remembering the 7 pillars is PIRATES

a. **P**atient experience and involvement—ensures patients and the public are involved in ideas and the development of services, e.g. via feedback forms, questionnaires and patient representatives on hospital boards.
b. **I**nformation technology—ensures that patient data is accurate and up to date. Confidentiality of data is maintained.
c. **R**isk management—having robust systems in place to monitor and minimize the risks to patients and staff. If mistakes or near misses occur, one should learn from them.
d. **A**udit—to ensure that clinical practice adheres to the current health standards.
e. **T**raining and education—essential for clinicians to keep up to date. This involves attending courses and conferences, taking relevant exams, workplace assessments and appraisals.
f. **C**linical **E**ffectiveness—ensuring that current clinical practice is designed to achieve the best outcome for patients. In practice, it means adopting an evidence-based approach, changing course if current practice is shown to be inadequate and conducting research to develop the body of evidence.
g. **S**taff management—ensures that the appropriate people are employed in the proper roles. Professional development of staff should be catered for.

 ## EVIDENCE-BASED MEDICINE

- **What is evidence-based medicine?**

  - It is the conscious, explicit and judicious use of current best evidence in making decisions about the care of individual patients. The practice of EBM means integrating individual clinical expertise with the best available clinical evidence from systematic research.

Steps involved in EBM:

1. Main question

2. Construct a clinical question from the main question that needs to be answered
3. Conduct research
4. Appraise evidence
5. Integrate evidence into practice to find a solution
6. Evaluate results

- **Why use clinical expertise in evidence-based medicine?**

  - The study/paper may be the best available regarding that topic; however, it may not be relevant to that patient.
  - Patients often have comorbidities that may influence clinical decision-making and may not be addressed fully in the papers being studied.

 TEACHING

- **What are the qualities of a good teacher?**

  - A good teacher is positive, supportive and encouraging and can enthuse students to want to learn. A good teacher will:

    a. Respect students
    b. Set appropriate goals
    c. Have a clear plan to achieve goals
    d. Involve students
    e. Can adapt their methods to the students
    f. Encourage feedback and develop further by reflecting on it

- **Why do you enjoy teaching?**

  - I enjoy helping colleagues/students learn about new ideas/techniques. It is particularly satisfying when students understand concepts that they previously found challenging.
  - I also find this to be a very effective learning tool for myself as I gain more insight into the topic by preparing and answering questions on it.

 TEAMWORK AND COMMUNICATION

- **What makes a good team player?**

  - Examples of this include someone who:
  - Understands their role in a team
  - Recognizes their duties and responsibilities
  - Appreciates the role of others in the team
  - Reliable and completes their work efficiently
  - Takes responsibility for their work
  - Aware of their limits and asks for help appropriately

- Communicates effectively with others
- Treats others with respect and courtesy
- Shows willingness to help others
- Listens to the concerns of colleagues
- Shows sensitivity toward colleagues
- Explains their thoughts clearly

 ## LEADERSHIP

- **What is leadership?**

  - Leadership is about having a vision and motivating people to achieve that goal or vision most effectively.
  - A leader can influence others, gaining the cooperation of others and create an environment where people can work together effectively.
  - A leader can achieve their targets by motivating their team. They can make decisions and apply knowledge to help them reach their goals. They also set their goals and targets by envisioning how the department or unit should develop in the future.

- **What makes a good leader?**

  - A good leader can motivate a team to achieve a goal using planning and delegation. They can have specific attributes—integrity, vision, support, effective communication, active listening and decision-making.

- **What is the difference between management and leadership?**

  - Leadership is about having a vision or setting a direction, whereas management is about controlling and coordinating resources in order to achieve the vision or direction set by the leader

Managers are reactive to others' ideas, whereas leaders seek to shape ideas.

SOME OF THE CHALLENGES FACING THE SURGEON TODAY

- Increased sub-specialization

  - General surgery is gradually being replaced by subspecialties. For the trainees, this can mean concentrated exposure to subspecialties so that it is relatively harder to gain a wider range of skills.

- Interventional radiology

  - Interventional radiology has changed the landscape in many specialties, more notably in vascular surgery. This is beneficial for patients; however, from a trainee's perspective, there are fewer cases for open surgery than before and the potential loss of associated skills.

- Robotic surgery

  - Robotic surgery is currently widely used in many surgical specialties such as colorectal and urology. It is more precise with associated smaller incisions and decreased blood loss, and it enables the surgeon to manipulate tissues in tiny spaces and on very small structures. This means that a whole new range of skills will be required, and certain specific skills may be degraded or lost, i.e. performing open operations.

- European Working Time Directive

  - This limits weekly working hours, which has its obvious advantages for work-life balance but unfortunately means that surgical trainees may not get enough hours of hands-on experience. In addition to this, it fragments the continuity of care, which means less follow-up of patients, e.g. taking history but not having the chance to go to theater and no longer finding the patient on the list the next day. Alternatively, going to theater to see a case but not knowing how they presented. It is worth noting that this legislative may be repealed in the future following the United Kingdom's recent departure from the European Union.

- The COVID-19 pandemic

  - This has limited training opportunities throughout all specialties. It has also created a massive backlog of surgical cases. In the future, there may be a higher number of service-provision operating lists with reduced time available for training purposes.

How to manage these challenges?

- Some of the examples include:

  1. Attending courses to expand on experience and learn new innovative skills such as in robotics to keep up with the changing surgical landscape.
  2. Simulation training—first pioneered by pilots in training and nowadays increasingly used in surgical teaching. Allows regular practice and development of skills in a safe and controlled environment. Most hospitals now have simulation laboratories.
  3. Seek support and advice from senior colleagues and mentors as there may be potential for greater exposure to operating lists and other helpful learning tools and activities.

2 Clinical Station

ABOUT THIS STATION

The clinical station is designed to assess your clinical knowledge and judgment and how you apply these to solve clinical problems.

Typically, you will be given a written clinical scenario, and you will be allocated a short period of time to read through the case and prepare your answer. You will be provided with a pen and paper to take notes. After the preparation time, you will enter the station, and you will be asked questions about the clinical scenario. The interviewers usually provide you with more information along the way and ask for further suggestions from management. The discussion may include additional topics related to the clinical case provided, which will be covered during the allotted time. Marks are awarded for the recognition of the clinical issues and use of clinical knowledge, judgment, prioritization and general communication in managing the case.

HOW TO TACKLE THIS STATION

1. Carefully read through the case provided and make sure that you have understood all the information provided.
2. You can make notes to help you structure your answer, preferably in bullet points. You must not spend too much time fussing over the notes, as this could potentially reduce your preparation time.
3. Have a system for answering the clinical question. This can then be applied to any clinical situation encountered. For example, your opening sentence should ideally summarize the clinical problem and identify the important issues that need to be addressed. You can also express what you are concerned about, e.g. *"Based on the information provided, I have a septic patient with suspected acute complicated appendicitis who requires expeditious resuscitation followed by definitive treatment."* You may also wish to begin with *"the key issue in this scenario is sepsis from a potentially complicated acute appendicitis which I would manage as follows..."* or *"This is clearly an emergency situation given the degree of sepsis which is likely due to acute complicated appendicitis and I would manage this as follows...."*
   Starting your answer as described will demonstrate to the interviewer that you have understood the clinical dilemma and have a plan of action to manage this case. Do not just repeat the full question back to the interviewer—this will reduce the time available for your answer and does not demonstrate any understanding on your part. It simply shows that you can repeat information!
4. When provided with more information and then asked a follow-up question, make sure you have understood the additional information that you have been given as this will shape your answer, e.g. the patient is 75 years old with moderate-to-severe chronic obstructive pulmonary disease and requires

DOI: 10.1201/9781003221739-2

an appendicectomy. What would be your approach, and why? The clue here is that the patient has a chronic respiratory disease. The consequence of this is that he might have impaired lung function and capacity and may not be able to tolerate the pneumoperitoneum if a laparoscopic approach was undertaken.

5. You will be provided with clinical scenarios taking place in different settings, for e.g. the unwell patient on the ward, the sick patient in A&E, a trauma call that may have been brought in (in some instances, "walked in")", or a patient in the clinic. Do not let this throw you off. In addition to your clinical knowledge and judgment, the interviewers are trying to gather evidence on your situational awareness.

The following is a format for how to tackle these specific clinical scenarios and examples of each. Each example here will take you through how to deliver the answer and contains suggested further reading relevant to the topic.

MANAGING THE SCENARIO OF THE "UNWELL PATIENT ON THE WARD" OR "UNWELL PATIENT IN A&E"

1. Use the **CCrISP** (Care of the Critically Ill Surgical Patient) outline to answer the question as follows:

    i. Assessment of Airway, Breathing, Circulation, Disability and Exposure (ABCDE) and resuscitation
    ii. Take a history, review any available operating notes and review the existing clinical notes
    iii. Examine the patient
    iv. Review the existing charts (observation, fluid balance, dug chart) and results (hematological, radiological)
    v. Decide whether the patient is STABLE or UNSTABLE based on the previous assessment
    vi. If stable, continue with management as follows . . .
    vii. If unstable, suggest additional investigations and a definitive treatment plan
    viii. Always update the patient, members of your team and the nursing staff about changes in management
    ix. Document your assessment and management plan clearly in the notes

CLINICAL SCENARIOS

 1. **The A&E team ask you to see a metastatic cancer patient (confirmed colorectal cancer with liver metastases) who is peritonitic, hypotensive and may have perforated. What do you do?**

Example of how to approach this answer:

    i. The issue here is that I have an unwell, septic patient with metastatic colorectal cancer who has a poor prognosis.

ii. I will want to gather more information while simultaneously resuscitating the patient before I make a final decision about definitive management.

iii. I will take the senior house officer (SHO) on call with me to review the patient to assist with the clinical management.

iv. I will manage this patient in concordance with the CCrISP protocol:

- Assess ABCDE and resuscitate the patient, ensuring the Sepsis 6 bundle is fully rolled out (sepsis 6 consists of oxygen, fluids, broad-spectrum antibiotics, take blood for investigations including lactate, take blood cultures and insert a urinary catheter)

- Take a history from the patient if the patient is able to provide a history and/or review the relevant clinic letters, in particular, noting:

  - The history of the cancer—when, where and how it was diagnosed.
  - The treatment the patient has received so far.
  - Cancer MDT discussions and outcomes and plans.
  - Ascertain whether the patient is aware of the progression of the disease.
  - The patient's pre-morbid status.
  - Any documented involvement of the palliative care team?
  - Any existing information on the ceiling of care if the patient deteriorated?
  - Any existing information on resuscitation status?

v. I will examine the patient and confirm the peritonitic status—localized or generalized peritonitis?

vi. I will then review the patient's observation chart, noting the degree of response to resuscitation and any available results such as blood or radiological results.

vii. I will need to confirm whether the patient is stabilizing or deteriorating.

- Given the information provided, it is probable that the patient is deteriorating; therefore, it is important at this stage to have a discussion with the patient and his or her family/Next-of-Kin about the possible management options which are:

  1. Major resectional surgery—the patient is unsuitable for this.
  OR
  2. Palliative, ward-based management.
  3. The final decision can be reached after considering the patient's background, current clinical status, American Society of Anesthesiology (ASA) grade and calculation of his PPOSSUM (Physiological and perioperative severity score for the enumeration of morbidity and mortality) score to predict his perioperative morbidity and mortality. A patient is deemed "high risk" if he or she has a predicted mortality on the PPOSSUM of > 5%. All patients

with a predicted perioperative mortality of >5% should have active consultant input and must be admitted to a critical care bed post-operatively, according to recommendations from the Royal College of Surgeons of England (RCS).

4. Patients with a mortality risk of 10% should only be managed under the direct supervision of a consultant surgeon and consultant anesthetist.

viii. In my opinion, this patient is not suitable for surgery and requires palliation, and I will consult the palliative care team.

ix. Palliative care or end-of-life pathway involves relief of symptoms such as pain, nausea, vomiting, discontinuation or alteration of certain medications and discontinuation of regular observations and interventions.

x. Discuss and document a resuscitation status.

- I will discuss and document a resuscitation status in the case of Cardio-pulmonary Arrest.
- I will involve my consultant early as this is a critically unwell patient, take my consultant through the background of the patient and the events thus far as well as my suggested plan for palliation.
- I will discuss the plan of management with the patient and involve the patient's family or Next-of-Kin.
- I will contact the palliative care team and transfer the patient to a side room.
- I will ensure that the events and various discussions have been fully documented.

 Suggested further reading

- CCrISP (Care of the Critically-ill Surgical Patient) management protocol
- Management of Septic shock
- Emergency presentations of colonic cancer and their management
- Palliative care and end-of-life pathways

 2. While you're on your way to the clinic, you get a call from one of the ward nurses regarding a patient who underwent an Abdominal Aortic Aneurysm (AAA) repair earlier that day. He has a painful, cold right leg, and she is concerned about possible lower limb ischemia. What would you do?

Example of how to approach this answer:

i. The issue here is that I have a clinic to do but an emergency on the ward has now come up in that a patient who is post AAA repair has suspected lower limb ischemia.

ii. I will advise the nurse over the phone to put the patient on high flow oxygen, place him nil-by-mouth and give him analgesia while I make my way to the ward.

   iii. I will inform my consultant and colleagues in the clinic about the ward emergency that has come up so that alternative cover can be sought or patients can be rescheduled if appropriate.

   iv. Once I get to the ward, I will review and manage the patient in concordance with the principles from the CCrISP protocol:

- Assessment of ABCDE and resuscitation, ensuring that the patient is put on high flow oxygen, opiate analgesia, intravenous fluids and large-bore intravenous access is gained. Immediate heparinization is required if a thrombus is suspected to prevent propagation of the occlusive thrombus.
- Take a history; review the operation note and the existing clinical notes. Ask about onset and duration of lower limb pain, any sensorimotor deficit, any prior history of claudication or arrhythmias, look at the details of the operation, noting any intra-operative technical difficulties and the time and length of the operation. The likely differential diagnoses are, if open aneurysm repair was undertaken, emboli from the disrupted plaque or new thrombus formation from diminished limb perfusion when the aortic clamp is on with subsequent embolization following clamp release. If an endovascular aortic repair (EVAR) approach was undertaken the possible causes may be graft limb kinking, access vessel injury such as thrombosis, dissection, pseudo-aneurysm and perforation.

- Examine the patient:

  - Carry out a full cardiovascular system's examination, examine the abdomen if open repair was performed, examine both groins if EVAR was undertaken. A hematoma at the operative site could raise a concern for a technical complication at the anastomosis and possible graft compression.
  - Examine the lower limbs

    - Inspect—pallor, blue discoloration, mottled, swelling
    - Palpate—temperature, pulses: proximal to distal
    - Doppler—proximal to distal

  - Review the existing charts (observation, fluid balance, urine output, drug chart) and any available results (hematological, radiological).

   v. In this case, the patient is clearly unwell with suspected acute lower limb ischaemia. Complete arterial occlusion will lead to irreversible tissue damage within six hours. He will require an urgent CT angiogram to establish the cause of the ischaemia followed by definitive management. Treatment of limb occlusion includes various surgical and endovascular revascularization techniques; the best treatment option will depend on the patient's general status as well as on local anatomic changes of the stent-graft. Examples include embolectomy if microemboli are suspected or endovascular adjustment of the graft if graft kinking is suspected.

   vi. Early involvement of the responsible consultant to plan definitive treatment.

vii. Update the patient, members of your team and the nursing staff about changes in management.

viii. Document clearly in the notes.

 Suggested further reading

- Complications following AAA repair
- Management of acute limb ischemia

 3. You are the ST3 on call, and you get a call from a triage nurse in A&E about a man with a swollen, red, painful scrotum with a pinpoint black area. You are in theater and about to do a laparoscopic appendicectomy. The patient is stable and awake with the anaesthetist.

Example of how to approach this answer:

i. The issues here are that there is a patient in A&E who may have Fournier's gangrene and requires urgent senior assessment and I'm also about to start a case in theater.

ii. I would start off by advising the triage nurse over the telephone to do the following:

- Get IV access and send of bloods for Full Blood Count (FBC), Urea and Electrolytes (UEs), C-reactive protein (CRP), blood cultures and Group and Screen (G&S).
- Move the patient to the Resuscitation bay.
- Get one of the senior A&E doctors to start reviewing the patient while I make plans for the case I currently have on the table.
- Inform the nurse that I will arrive within 15 minutes.

iii. Next, I would inform the anesthetist about the emergency that a life-threatening emergency has come up and request that he/she does not anesthetize the appendicectomy case. I would inform my consultant of this delay to the operation. The appendicectomy patient is stable, and therefore their operation could potentially wait until I have reviewed the patient with suspected Fournier's gangrene. Additionally, the patient with suspected Fournier's gangrene may need to be brought to theater for surgery as a priority ahead of the appendicectomy case. Fournier's gangrene is a necrotizing fasciitis of the perineum caused by synergistic infection with aerobic and anaerobic organisms. It can rapidly progress to severe sepsis, multi-organ failure and death if there is a delay in treatment.

iv. I will promptly go to A&E Resus and manage the patient following the principles of CCrISP:

- Assess ABCDE and resuscitate the patient, ensuring the Sepsis 6 bundle is fully rolled out (sepsis 6: oxygen, fluids, broad-spectrum

antibiotics, take bloods including lactate, take blood cultures and insert
urinary catheter). Test the blood glucose and perform a urine analysis.

- Take a history and examine the patient, particularly checking for a history of diabetes mellitus, recent localized infection, trauma to the genitalia and fully examine the scrotum and genitalia, perineum, abdomen, thigh and buttocks specifically looking for cellulitic changes, dusky blue or black skin suggestive of underlying necrosis, abscesses, palpable crepitus. Assess for systemic features of sepsis or severe sepsis.
- Review available results which often demonstrate raised inflammatory markers, acidaemia, impaired renal function, impaired clotting.
- If the findings suggest Fournier's gangrene, the patient needs urgent surgical debridement. The diagnosis is entirely clinical. Early surgical debridement is paramount and if delayed will have adversely impact the patient's prognosis. I will then proceed as follows:

vi. Inform the consultant surgeon on call.
vii. Inform the anaesthetic and emergency theater staff to make prompt arrangements for surgery.
viii. Prepare the patient for surgery with consenting and marking if applicable.
ix. Discuss the case with the intensive care team as the patient will most likely require a critical care bed post-operatively.
x. The principles of surgery are debridement of all necrotic and nonviable tissue however extensive, make arrangements for a return to theater in 24 hours for further reassessment and/or +/- debridement.

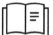 **Suggested further reading**

- Necrotizing fasciitis

 4. You are the On-call Surgical Registrar, and at 6 pm, you are called to the main surgical ward by the nurse in charge to review a 45-year-old woman who was re-admitted overnight with worsening abdominal pain, 4 days following laparoscopic appendicectomy. The day team had arranged a CT scan for her which didn't happen till 5 pm. The report has just come back demonstrating a retained surgical swab.

Example of how to approach this answer:

i. The main issue here is that the patient has a retained swab which not only has led to the patient being septic, but it is also a serious incident and a never event.
ii. I would promptly go to the ward and assess the patient.
iii. I would manage the patient following the principles of CCrISP:

- Assess ABCDE and resuscitate her, ensuring the Sepsis 6 bundle is fully rolled out if this hasn't been started already. The sepsis 6 are supplementing the patient with high-flow oxygen, ensuring that the patient has intravenous fluids running and that she is on broad-spectrum antibiotics in concordance with the Trust's anti-microbial protocol. I would ensure that she has had blood tests, including a lactate profile, blood cultures and a urinary catheter inserted.

- Next, I would take a focused history from the patient and review the existing clinical notes, in particular the operation note and her clinical course and management since then.
- I would examine the patient and review her observation chart as well as fluid balance and drug charts.
- I would review all available clinical results and carefully review the CT images to identify the size and site of the retained swab, any associated collections, any suspicion of iatrogenic injury and I would discuss any queries with the radiologist.

iv. The patient will require an operation to remove the retained swab which is the source of the sepsis. I will discuss the case and the management plan with the consultant on call. However, ahead of this, the patient will need to be informed of the findings. This is likely to cause distress to the patient, so it is important that I handle the matter sensitively.

v. As per the duty of candor, I will talk to the patient with the nurse in charge present and will document the discussion and management plan carefully.

vi. I will consent the patient for laparoscopic and/or open removal of retained swab and liaise with the emergency theater and anesthetic team to plan the timing of surgery.

vii. I would complete an incident form and ensure that the case is added to the next morbidity and mortality meeting for discussion.

viii. I would offer the patient support and respect her wishes to make a complaint and advise her of the formal complaints process.

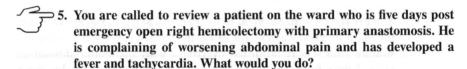

5. You are called to review a patient on the ward who is five days post emergency open right hemicolectomy with primary anastomosis. He is complaining of worsening abdominal pain and has developed a fever and tachycardia. What would you do?

Example of how to approach this answer:

i. The main issue here is that the patient is unwell and displaying features of sepsis five days following emergency colectomy. My primary concern would be an anastomotic leak until I can prove otherwise.

ii. I would promptly go to the ward and assess the patient.

iii. I would manage the patient following the principles of CCrISP:

- Assess ABCDE and resuscitate him, ensuring the Sepsis 6 bundle is fully rolled out. The sepsis 6 are supplementing the patient with high-flow oxygen, ensuring that the patient has intravenous fluids running and that he is started on broad-spectrum antibiotics in concordance with the Trust's anti-microbial protocol. I would ensure that he has had blood tests including a lactate profile, blood cultures and a urinary catheter inserted. He also requires an ECG given the tachyarrhythmia.

- Next, I would take a focused history from the patient and review the existing clinical notes, in particular the operation note and his clinical course and management since then. From this I would want to ascertain the following:

  - The indication for the emergency right hemicolectomy and intra-operative findings such as peritoneal soiling or contamination.
  - The patient's clinical course since the operation, including level of pain and analgesic requirements, trend in observation and blood results, oral intake, bowel function, overall progress.
  - The patient's background and existing medical comorbidities.
  - The patient's current symptoms, specifically to ascertain if there could be other sources of sepsis; when did the abdominal pain become worse? Any pain or swelling around wound sites? Any respiratory symptoms? Any urinary symptoms? Any features of infection around intravenous lines? Any calf pain? N.B.: aide memoir to causes of post-op fever: 6Cs (Chest, Catheter, Cut, Cannula, CVP line and Calf for deep vein thrombosis).

- I would examine the patient's abdomen and chest, and review his observation chart as well as fluid balance and drug charts.
- I would review all available results including the most recent blood results and any urine tests or chest X-rays.
- At this stage, my impression is that I have an unwell patient in whom I need to exclude an anastomotic leak. *Any disturbance in physiology in a patient with a new bowel anastomosis is a leak until proven otherwise.*
- Alongside full resuscitation, I would arrange for the patient to have an urgent CT scan of the abdomen and pelvis to look for an anastomotic leak or collections.
- I would contact the on-call radiologist to discuss the case in order to expedite the CT scan.
- I would contact the consultant on call and responsible consultant to give them an update on the patient and my plan of management.
- I would inform the patient and nursing staff of the plan and keep the patient nil-by-mouth.
- I would ensure that the clinical assessment and full plan are documented clearly in the notes as well as a plan for review with the results to plan the next step in management.

A follow-up question might be: What are the risk factors for an anastomotic leak and how would you manage a leak in this scenario?

i. The risk factors for a leak may be general patient factors (advanced age, frailty, malnutrition, immunosuppression, anemia, uremia, smoking) or specific related to the surgery (anastomosis under tension, ischemia of the tissues, infection/cross-contamination).
ii. The management depends on whether the leak is localized or generalized and the general condition of the patient.

- Localized leak:
  Conservative management with bowel rest, parenteral nutrition and antibiotics. A collection of pus around the anastomosis can be drained percutaneously under USS or CT guidance if >5 cm.
- Generalized peritonitis:
  Optimize the hemodynamic status of the patient followed by surgical management; extensive lavage of peritoneal cavity and either

  1. Take the anastomosis apart and exteriorize as an end stoma and mucus fistula
     or
  2. In selected patients, if the defect is small, it may be possible to repair it and construct a defunctioning ileostomy to divert away from the area of the leak. Carry out transanal irrigation to prevent continued soiling.

 Suggested further reading

- Anastomotic dehiscence
- Post-operative causes of sepsis

MANAGING THE SCENARIO OF A "TRAUMA CALL"

1. Use the ATLS outline (Advanced Trauma Life Support)

   i. Ensure a trauma call was put out if it hasn't happened already.
   ii. Take a junior member of the team with you to review the patient.
   iii. If the patient is in another area of A&E, move the patient to resuscitation bay.
   iv. Conduct the primary survey with simultaneous resuscitation.

   a. **Airway maintenance with restriction of cervical spine motion:** ensure adequate airway, i.e. ability to speak clearly/ability to generate air movement to facilitate speech and C-spine immobilization (collar, blocks and tape)—assume that a spinal injury exists until proven otherwise.
   b. **Breathing and ventilation:** assess respiratory rate, oxygen saturation, position of the trachea, distension of jugular veins, inspect/palpate/percuss/auscultate chest, apply high flow O_2.
   c. **Circulation with hemorrhage control:** assess pulse rate, blood pressure, signs of shock and visible hemorrhage, listen to heart sounds, identify source of hemorrhage as internal or external, gain large-bore intravenous access and appropriate replacement of intravascular volume, send blood tests.
   d. **Disability (neurological evaluation):** perform Glasgow Coma Scale assessment to establish the patient's level of consciousness, pupillary size and reaction and to identify any lateralizing signs. Check the blood glucose.

e. **Exposure and environmental control:** expose fully for a full examination. After completing the assessment, cover the patient with blankets or an external warming device to prevent hypothermia.

f. **Adjuncts to the primary survey:** Continuous electrocardiography, pulse oximetry, arterial blood gas, carbon dioxide (CO_2) monitoring or capnography—a non-invasive monitoring technique that assesses end-tidal CO_2 levels in order to provide information on the patient's ventilation, a urinary catheter (reflects renal perfusion and indicator of patient's volume status), gastric tube (decompressed stomach and reduces the risk of aspiration), X-ray examinations (AP chest, AP pelvis)—do obtain essential X-ray examinations even in pregnant women, Focussed Assessment with Sonography in Trauma (FAST), eFAST (extended Focussed Assessment with Sonography in Trauma) and Diagnostic Peritoneal Lavage (DPL) for quick detection of free intra-abdominal fluid, pneumothorax or hemothorax.

v.   **Conduct the secondary survey—once the primary survey is completed and resuscitative efforts are underway**.

a. **Head-to-toe examination**—complete history and physical examination including reassessment of all the vital signs (will repeat some examinations already undertaken in the primary survey and will be further informed by the progress of the resuscitation).

b. **Adjuncts to the secondary survey:** specialized diagnostic tests to look for specific injuries: additional XRs of the limbs or extremities, CT scan of the head, chest, abdomen and spine, contrast angiography or urn graphs, transesophageal ultrasound, endoscopy, bronchoscopy.

CLINICAL SCENARIOS

 1. **A 14-year-old boy is brought into A&E by his father with left upper quadrant pain after striking his abdomen against his bicycle's handlebar. They have only just arrived in triage. You are the on-call surgical registrar and you were about to head back to the office after reviewing a patient. What would you do?**

Example of how to approach this answer:

i. This is a case of trauma, and currently, there is uncertainty about the extent of injury. However, given the mechanism, I'd be particularly concerned about a splenic injury.

ii. I would get the patient into the resuscitation bay, and I would put out a trauma call.

iii. Once the members of the trauma team arrive, which should be within minutes, I would lead the trauma call by assigning individuals to their roles and following the principles of ATLS.

iv. I would start with the primary survey as follows:

- Airway and C-spine immobilization: ensure adequate airway by assessing if the patient can speak and immobilize the C-spine with collar, blocks and tape.
- Breathing and ventilation—assess respiratory rate, oxygen saturations, position of the trachea, examine chest: inspect for bruising particularly on the left side and how the chest is rising with respiration, palpate for swelling/crepitus, percuss for hyper-resonant or dull sounds that could indicate pneumothorax or hemothorax, respectively, auscultate for breath sounds comparing right and left sides, put the patient on 15 L of O_2 with a non-rebreather mask.
- Circulation and hemorrhage control—assess patient's pulse, blood pressure, look for signs of shock (pallor, cool peripheries, delayed capillary refill time), listen to the chest for heart sounds, get bilateral large-bore intravenous access and use this opportunity to send off the following blood tests: Full Blood Count/Urea and Eelectrolytes/cross-match 4 units. Examine the abdomen looking for bruising around the left side and focal points of tenderness, start administration of warm fluids (in trauma, 1L crystalloid rapid bolus or 10–20 mL/kg in children), provide analgesia.
- Disability—assess the patient's Glasgow Coma Scale (GCS) and test blood glucose.
- Exposure—expose the patient fully and actively look for other associated or distracting injuries

Adjuncts to primary survey

- Adjuncts that I would consider in this case: Arterial Blood Gas, trauma series XRs and a FAST scan to assess for free fluid in the abdomen, particularly around the region of the spleen.

  v. I would then carry out the secondary survey with a complete history about the details of the incident and the symptoms the patient has: e.g. left upper quadrant pain and left should tip pain may be caused by diaphragmatic irritation due to subdiaphragmatic bleeding; this is known as Kehr's sign. I would carry out a full head-to-toe examination to pick up any other missed injuries. This would also involve reassessment of vital signs to assess response to resuscitation. If the patient is now hemodynamically stable, I would obtain a contrast-enhanced CT scan of the chest, abdomen, pelvis, looking specifically for injuries on the left side of the chest such as pneumothorax, hemothorax, flail segment, pulmonary contusion and a splenic injury.

 vi. If the patient is unstable despite full resuscitation and there is a concern for active hemorrhage from an injured spleen, the patient will require an operation to control the hemorrhage. I will immediately inform the on-call consultant and will make arrangements for theater for an exploratory laparotomy.

vii. I would speak to the on-call anesthetist and theater coordinator and get the patient booked and consented for surgery. The patient is 15 years old, and if he is deemed Gillick competent, then he can sign the consent form. A child under the age of 16 years is deemed Gillick competent if he or she can understand, retain and weigh up the information in terms of risks and benefits. Even if a child is competent, every effort should be made to encourage the child to involve their parents.

A follow-up question might be: How do you grade splenic trauma?

- Grading is done using the American Association of Surgery in Trauma classification which grades the injury based on the **depth of laceration** and the **extent of associated hematoma:**

  Grade 1 depth <1 cm, hematoma <10%
  Grade 2 depth 1–3 cm, hematoma 10%–50%
  Grade 3 depth >3 cm, hematoma >50%
  Grade 4 involvement of hilar/segmental vessels
  Grade 5 shattered spleen

A second follow-up question might be: summarize for me how these injuries are managed.

- 1–3 can be managed conservatively (close observation and bed rest, serial abdominal examination and Hb check every 6 hours and/or angio-embolization if CT shows contrast blush or extravasation)
- 4–5 require splenectomy

A third follow-up question might be: what is the management following emergency splenectomy?

- Vaccinations: meningococcal, pneumococcal, Hemophilus influenza type B as soon as possible post-emergency splenectomy, ideally within 2 weeks (following splenectomy, these organisms will not be phagocytosed)
- Yearly influenza vaccination
- Lifelong Penicillin V
- Medical bracelet stating asplenic status
- Activity restriction for three months

 2. **You are the ST3 in general surgery at a district general hospital. You are called to A&E as part of a trauma call for a 23-year-old male who has suffered a stab wound to the left side of his chest. When you arrive, he is very anxious and has saturations of 94% on 4 L, a pulse rate of 120 bpm and a blood pressure of 75/60. There is no tracheal deviation, but you notice that he has grossly distended neck veins. The trauma team that has been assembled includes an anesthetic SHO, A&E registrar and the surgery FY2. How would you proceed?**

Example of how to approach this answer:

i. This is a case of penetrating left-sided chest trauma and the possible organs that could be injured are the heart, the great vessels, the left lung and pleura, the diaphragm and possibly intra-abdominal organs such as the spleen, stomach and left lobe of the liver.

ii. Given the vital parameters provided, the main differentials are cardiac tamponade or hemothorax.

iii. A trauma call has been put out and the trauma team have assembled. I would lead the trauma call, following the principles of ATLS.

iv. I would start with the primary survey as follows:

- Airway and C-spine immobilization: ensure adequate airway by talking to the patient and assessing if he can speak and immobilize the C-spine with collar, blocks and tape.
- Breathing and ventilation—the patient has low oxygen saturations, and I would also check his respiratory rate. The trachea is central which most likely excludes a tension pneumothorax. I would examine his chest by assessing the stab wound site and covering it with a sterile dressing, assessing the movement of the chest with respiration, checking whether the left hemithorax is hyper-resonant or dull to percussion if there is good air entry and breath sounds or if they are absent. Tension pneumothorax particularly on the left side can mimic cardiac tamponade. The presence of hyper-resonance on percussion indicates tension pneumothorax, whereas the presence of bilateral breath sounds in this case points more toward cardiac tamponade. I would put the patient on 15 L of O_2 with a non-rebreather mask.
- Circulation and haemorrhage control: the patient is tachycardic, hypotensive and has distended neck veins. I would listen to his heart, and if the heart sounds are muffled, then this points to a diagnosis of cardiac tamponade. The classic triad of muffled heart sounds, distended jugular veins and hypotension is known as Beck's triad and is pathognomonic for cardiac tamponade but is not uniformly present.
  I would get bilateral large-bore IV access and use this opportunity to send off the following blood tests: Full Blood Count/Urea and Electrolytes/cross-match four units.
- Disability—assess the patient's GCS and test blood glucose
- Exposure—expose the patient fully and actively look for any other associated or distracting injuries
- At this stage, my primary differential is cardiac tamponade. My primary adjunct to confirm this diagnosis is a FAST scan which is a rapid and accurate bedside test for imaging the heart and pericardium. It is 90%–95% accurate at identifying the presence of pericardial fluidic experienced hands. I would ask the A&E registrar to perform this.
- If it confirms cardiac tamponade, the most up-to-date ATLS guidance is to undertake emergency thoracotomy by a qualified emergency physician or surgeon as soon as possible. If trained personnel are not immediately available, then pericardiocentesis, preferably with ultrasound guidance, is used as a temporizing measure until a thoracotomy can be undertaken.

- Once the cardiac tamponade is treated fully and full reassessment of the primary survey is undertaken, the secondary head-to-toe survey can be undertaken.
- I would ensure that I update my consultant about the case and document all aspects of it clearly.
- I would consider the need for tetanus immunization if the patient is not fully immunized.

  A follow-up question might be: What is the pathophysiology of cardiac tamponade?

- Cardiac tamponade occurs when the heart is compressed by external pressure from fluid accumulation in the pericardial sac. The pericardial sac is a rigid fibrous structure which does not expand well. Even a relatively small volume of blood within this sac could restrict cardiac filling and function. It most commonly occurs from penetrating injuries.

  A second follow-up question might be: How do the signs in Beck's triad manifest in cardiac tamponade?

- Muffled heart sounds—due to blood or clot around the heart muffling the sounds of the valve closures.
- Distended jugular veins—due to impaired diastolic filling of the right atrium.
- Hypotension—due to impaired cardiac function and low cardiac output.

 3. A 45-year-old woman fell off a tall ladder while doing some work in her garden. She is complaining of severe right-sided abdominal pain. On arrival in A&E Resus, she is tachycardia but normotensive with bruising around the right side of her abdomen. How would you manage this patient?

Example of how to approach this answer:

i. This is a case of blunt trauma to the right chest and abdomen and the possible organs that could be injured are the left lung and pleura, the diaphragm and intra-abdominal solid organs such as the liver.

ii. I would get the patient into the resuscitation bay, and I would put out a trauma call.

iii. Once the members of the trauma team arrive, which should be within minutes, I would lead the trauma call by assigning individuals to their roles and following the principles of ATLS.

iv. I would start with the primary survey as follows:

- Airway and C-spine immobilization: ensure adequate airway by talking to the patient and assessing if she can speak and immobilize the C-spine with collar, blocks and tape.
- Breathing and ventilation—I would assess her respiratory rate and oxygen saturation. I would assess the position of the trachea and examine her chest, inspecting for bruising/swelling/open wounds, palpating for fractures ribs and assessing the movement of the chest

with respiration. I would percuss for hyper-resonant or dull sounds that could indicate pneumothorax or hemothorax, respectively, and I would auscultate for breath sounds comparing right and left sides. At this stage, I would put the patient on 15 L of O_2 with a non-rebreather mask.

- Circulation and hemorrhage control—although she is normotensive, she is tachycardic, which could be because she is in severe pain or she may have grade 2 hypovolemic shock which would suggest underlying hemorrhage. I would confirm that she has shock by assessing for additional features such as pallor, coolness of peripheries and delayed capillary refill time. I would listen to the chest for heart sounds, get bilateral large-bore intravenous access and use this opportunity to send off the following blood tests: Full Blood Count/Urea and Electrolytes/cross-match 4 units. I would examine the abdomen and assess for peritonism. I would assess for other potential sites for hemorrhage such as the pelvis, long bones and open hemorrhaging wounds. I would administer warm fluids and provide analgesia.
- Disability—assess the patient's GCS and test blood glucose.
- Exposure—expose the patient fully and actively look for other associated or distracting injuries.

- I would then carry out the secondary survey with a complete history about the details of the incident and conduct a full head-to-toe examination. This would also involve reassessment of vital signs to assess response to resuscitation. If the patient has responded well to resuscitation and remains hemodynamically stable, I would obtain a contrast-enhanced CT scan of the chest, abdomen and pelvis.
- The interviewer may follow up with: The CT scan demonstrates a 3 cm laceration in segment 8 of the liver with a surrounding hematoma. There is no extravasation of contrast seen. His Hb comes back as 112 g/L. How would you manage this patient?

  - The patient has sustained a liver laceration, but given that she is hemodynamically stable and there is no active bleeding and no significant anemia, I would manage her conservatively. This involves admission to a high dependency unit, strict bed rest, close observation of vital parameters and daily bloods to assess for a drop in hemoglobin and her liver function tests.

A follow-up question might be: If on day 2 her Hb dropped to 78 g/L and her abdominal pain got worse, what would be the treatment then?

- This would signify further and likely active bleeding that requires a further intervention which might be in the form of radiological treatment or surgical intervention.
- These cases should ideally be managed in tertiary centre with the expertise for dealing with liver trauma.

4. **You are the on-call surgical registrar and you are called to A&E to a 50-year-old man in Resus. He was the driver of a car that was involved in a high-speed collision into the back of a stationary vehicle. He is tachypnoeic and hypoxic with saturations of 91% on room air. He has a pulse of 115 bpm and a blood pressure of 90/50. How would you proceed?**

Example of how to approach this answer:

i. This is a case of significant deceleration trauma, and there may be a multitude of injuries.

ii. I would get the patient into the resuscitation bay, and I would put out a trauma call.

iii. Once the members of the trauma team arrive, which should be within minutes, I would lead the trauma call by assigning individuals to their roles and following the principles of ATLS.

iv. I would start with the primary survey as follows:

- Airway and C-spine immobilization—ensure adequate airway by talking to the patient and assessing if he is able to speak and immobilizes the C-spine with collar, blocks and tape.

- Breathing and ventilation—the patient is tachypnoeic with low saturations, and in this situation, I would suspect trauma to the chest. I would assess the position of the trachea. If it is deviated, then this could suggest a tension pneumothorax. I would examine his chest, inspecting for bruising/swelling/open wounds around the chest wall. I would palpate for fractures ribs/flail segments and assess the movement of the chest with respiration. I would percuss for hyper-resonant or dull sounds that could indicate pneumothorax or hemothorax, respectively, and I would auscultate for breath sounds comparing right and left sides to assess if they are equal. At this stage, I would put the patient on 15 L of O_2 with a non-rebreather mask.

- Circulation and hemorrhage control—the patient is shocked given the tachycardia and hypotension. With the mechanism involved, I would suspect hemorrhage, with the most likely source being the chest given his associated tachypnoea and low saturations. However, I would also assess for other potential sites for hemorrhage such as the abdomen, pelvis, long bones and open hemorrhaging wounds. I would listen to the heart sounds. I would obtain bilateral large-bore IV access and use this opportunity to send off the following blood tests: FBC/UEs/crossmatch 4 units. I would examine the abdomen and assess for peritonism, and I would administer warm fluids and provide analgesia.

- Disability—assess the patient's GCS and test blood glucose.

- Exposure—expose the patient fully and actively look for other associated or distracting injuries.

- At this stage, you may be told that the breath sounds in the right chest were absent and there was dullness to percussion.

- The most likely diagnosis at this stage is a massive haemeothorax which is suggested by the state of shock in association with absence of breath sounds and dullness to percussion on the right side of the chest. I would confirm this by obtaining a chest X-ray which would confirm the diagnosis by demonstrating blunting of the costophrenic angle or partial or complete opacification of the right side of the thorax.
- The patient will require decompression of the right chest cavity with a chest drain (size 28–32 French). Using an aseptic technique, I would insert the chest drain in the fifth intercostal space just anterior to the midaxillary line. I would also commence a transfusion of O negative or type-specific blood as soon as possible.
- I would monitor how much blood is draining out of the chest drain. The immediate drain of 1500 mL or more of blood is generally an indication for thoracotomy.
- Once the chest drain is positioned and transfusion is underway, I would go back to the start of the primary surgery and reassess the patient.
- Once the primary survey is completed, I would move on to the secondary survey with a complete history and I would conduct a full head-to-toe examination.
- The patient was involved in a high-speed collision and may well have other associated injuries, which I would need to look for.
- Once the patient has stabilized, he will most likely require a full-body CT scan.

  A follow-up question might be: What are the indications for thoracotomy in a case of a hemothorax?
- Immediate return of 1500 mL or more of blood after chest drain insertion.
- A rate of continued blood loss of 200 mL/hour for 2–4 hours.
- Persistent need for blood transfusion which indicates continued blood loss.

 Suggested further reading

How to perform emergency thoracotomy

 5. **You are at a trauma call as the surgical registrar where a 17-year-old boy was attacked earlier today and sustained a stab wound in the region of the left upper quadrant/lower chest. He is in respiratory distress with oxygen saturation that has been steadily dropping, now at 82% on room air. His shirt has been removed and you notice that the left side of his chest is not moving with respiration. What would you do?**

Example of how to approach this answer:

i. This is a case of penetrating trauma, with my immediate concern being a tension pneumothorax given the parameters provided. However, I would also warn to exclude other life-threatening injuries such as cardiac tamponade.

ii. I would lead the trauma call by assigning individuals to their roles and following the principles of ATLS.

iii. I would start with the primary survey as follows:

- Airway and C-spine immobilization—ensure adequate airway by talking to the patient and assessing if he is able to speak and immobilize the C-spine with collar, blocks and tape.
- Breathing and ventilation—the patient is in respiratory distress with saturations that are gradually dropping and the left side of his chest in not moving. I would assess the position of the trachea, and if it is deviated to the right, this would highly suggest a tension pneumothorax. This is confirmed by a hyper-resonant percussion note and absence of breath sounds on auscultation of the left hemithorax. Tension pneumothorax develops when a "one-way" valve air leak occurs from the lung to the pleura (visceral pleural injury). This allows gas to escape from the lung into the pleural space with every inspiration, but it cannot escape, eventually collapsing the affected lung. The mediastinum is displaced to the opposite side, decreasing venous return and eventually compressing the opposite lung. This is a clinical diagnosis, and I would not delay treatment by obtaining radiological confirmation.
- Before proceeding any further, I would proceed with immediate decompression with a large bore cannula or over-the-needle catheter into the fifth intercostal space just anterior to the midaxillary line. If the chest wall is thick and needle decompression is not successful, I would use my finger to perform finger thoracostomy. This will convert a tension pneumothorax into a simple pneumothorax. Tube or chest drain thoracostomy is mandatory after needle or finger decompression of the chest.
- Once the patient has a chest drain in, I will go back to Airway and then Breathing assessment. Only once I am satisfied with this, I will proceed with circulation and hemorrhage control, disability, exposure and the secondary survey.
- A follow-up question might be: Talk to me through the steps of placement of a chest drain.
  NB: Anytime you are asked to describe a procedure, use the 4Ps method to structure your answer: preparation, positioning, procedure, post-procedure plan
- Preparation—obtain verbal consent, ensure the site is marked, ensure all equipment needed is available (sizes 28–32 French chest drain, underwater seal container and tube, fast-acting local anaesthetic such as lignocaine 1%, scalpel, artery forceps, betadine or chlorhexidine skin prep, sterile gloves).
- Positioning—patient sitting up at 45-degree angle with arm on affected side behind head.
- Procedure—drain is sited in the "triangle of safety—edge of pectoralis major, mid axillary line, between second and fifth intercostal spaces. Infiltrate local anesthesia and mark point of entry (fifth intercostal space just anterior to mid-axillary line). Prepare the area

using antiseptic skin preparation. Make a 2 cm transverse incision along the upper border of the rib to avoid the neurovascular bundle. Use blunt dissection itch artery forceps to go through the layers of the intercostal muscles down to the pleural cavity, Insert a finger through the tract and sweep it around to clear the lung. Insert the chest drain, guiding it with the forceps. Drains for air should be placed towards the apex and anterior, whereas drains for fluid should be placed basally and posterior. Secure the drain using a purse-string suture.

- Post-procedure care—CXR to check drain placement is correct. Monitor drain output and perform regular drain checks for swinging and air leaks.

MANAGING THE SCENARIO OF A "PATIENT IN CLINIC"

1. Gather information before you start the consultation.

   i. NEW or FOLLOW-UP—if follow-up, how many prior attendances for the same problem.
   ii. Urgency of referral—routine, urgent, two-week wait.
   iii. Review the clinical information available such as past clinic letters, Multi-disciplinary team (MDT) discussion outcomes.
   iv. Review any available results.

2. Review patient and assess patient clinically.
3. Discuss findings and the full plan of management.
4. Assess patient's understanding of the situation and answer any relevant questions.
5. Plan and discuss follow-up.

CLINICAL SCENARIOS

 1. A 28-year-old patient came to the clinic as an urgent referral for recent-onset fresh rectal bleeding and mucus. He has a family history of colonic cancer. He had a recent colonoscopy organized by his GP in the lead up to the clinic appointment.

Example of how to approach this answer:

   i. I can see that this is a new, urgent referral with lower gastrointestinal symptoms.
   ii. Before I bring the patient into the clinic room, I would like to check the following:

   - Any prior clinic consultations with similar presentation?
   - Any attendances to A&E with this problem?
   - Any other information from the GP letter or other letters about the family history of colonic cancer? Any mention of family history of inflammatory bowel disease?
   - How recent is the colonoscopy and what does it show?—I would review pictures taken at the time and the full report.

- Any biopsies taken and the results of those?
- Any blood or stool results?

iii. I would then bring the patient into the clinic room and take a full history, enquiring specifically about:

- Onset and duration of fresh rectal bleeding
- Colour of the blood and estimate of volume
- Painful or painless bleeding
- Any associated perianal lumps or itching
- Any change in bowel habit
- Any weight-loss
- Any constitutional symptoms such as fever/malaise
- Past medical history, drug history, surgical history
- Full details of family history of colon cancer—number of relatives, first/second/third degree, age when cancer diagnosis was made. Any family history of inflammatory bowel disease

iv. I would then conduct a full examination including Digital Rectal Examination and proctosigmoidoscopy.

v. I would discuss any positive findings with the patient and plan any further investigations.

vi. I would assess patient's understanding of the situation and answer any questions.

vii. I would arrange appropriate follow-up.

 Suggested further reading

- Hereditary colorectal cancer syndromes
- Inflammatory bowel disease

 2. A 40-year-old woman with learning difficulties comes to the colorectal clinic with a Carer. She had been complaining of intermittent RUQ pin for many months. Recent blood tests demonstrated mildly deranged liver function tests in an obstructive profile three months earlier, which have recently returned to normal. How will you manage her?

Example of how to approach this answer:

i. The issue here is that I have a patient with learning difficulties who sounds like she may have symptomatic gallstones and may have recently passed a common bile duct stone.

ii. Before I bring the patient in, I would review the clinical notes to assess if there is a known history of gallstone disease and any previous hospital presentations or admissions with these symptoms.

iii. I would review her liver function tests and the rest of her blood results such as White Cell Count, C-Reactive Protein, Amylase and any previous scans the patient may have had.

iv. I would then bring her into the clinic with her Carer and advocate and review the history:

- Onset and duration of the pain, any exacerbating or relieving factors, any associated symptoms such as vomiting, fever, malaise and any history of jaundice.
- Any previous biliary surgery or biliary interventions, any other medical history and drug history.
- Social history—assess type and severity of learning disability and obtain information of information on support and care package and the patient's quality of life—get statements from Carer.
- Ask if the patient has a Next-Of-Kin (NOK) or Independent Mental Capacity Advocate (IMCA).
- I would then examine the patient with the help of a Carer, looking for general signs such as jaundice, pyrexia, dehydration, focal points of tenderness, Murphy's sign and Charcot's triad.
- I would also assess the patient's capacity for consent (1—able to understand information? 2—Able to weigh up risks and benefits and understand alternatives? 3—Able to retain information? 4—Able to make a decision without duress?)
  You are told that the patient had an ultrasound scan three days ago which demonstrated small gallstones and a normal calibre common bile duct. What is your next step in management, assuming that the patient has no NOK?
- It sounds like the patient may have passed a small stone when her liver function tests were deranged three months earlier. They have now normalized and her common bile duct is of normal caliber; therefore, there is no indication for any further imaging of the biliary tree or endoscopic retrograde cholangiopancreatography (ERCP).
- However, she will require a laparoscopic cholecystectomy.
- She has learning disabilities and therefore may not have capacity to consent.
- I would formally assess her capacity as described earlier and involve a clinical psychologist or psychiatrist for formal assessment of capacity if there is any doubt about her capacity.
- Since she has no NOK, it is important that I involve an IMCA to help with the patient's understanding of the situation and assist with the consent process since a cholecystectomy is in her best interest if she is surgically fit.
- I would document all discussions and enclose copies of statements from her Carer and the IMCA.
  A follow-up question might be: Give me examples of situations where formal assessment of capacity is required:

1. If a patient has a mental illness or learning disabilities
2. When the patient has made a decision that seems unwise or irrational
3. When capacity fluctuates
4. When the decision about the patient's capacity has or is likely to be challenged by a friend, relative or advocate

- The **Mental Capacity Act of 2005** allows for formal capacity assessments to be done by individuals such as clinical psychologists or psychiatrists
- Must have a "reasonable belief" backed by objective reasons that a patient lacks capacity
- Where there are disputes about an individual's lack of capacity, the **Court of Protection** can be asked for a judgment
- All decisions taken on behalf of someone who lacks capacity must be taken in his or her best interest unless they have an advanced directive A follow-up question might be: What is an IMCA and what is their role?
- An IMCA is an Independent Mental Capacity Advocate
- They support vulnerable adults who lack capacity to make certain decisions where there are no family members available or willing to be consulted about those decisions
- IMCAs advise, clarify and enable a person with a learning disability to make a decision
- An IMCA cannot be instructed if an individual has previously named a person who should be consulted about decisions that affect them

 3. **A 24-year-old woman has come to the clinic with recurrent boils in her groins and axilla. She has already undergone three incision and drainage operations. How will you manage her?**

Example of how to approach this answer:

i. This patient sounds like she has hydradenitis supprativa given her history of recurrent boils.
ii. Before I bring the patient in, I would review the clinical notes, ascertaining the number of admissions the patient has had related to this, number of operations, last operation, whether she has been referred to dermatology.
iii. I would bring the patient in and take a history; onset of history of boils, sites affected, check whether she had surgeries or consultations in other hospitals, antibiotic use, whether she is a smoker, any history of diabetes mellitus or if this has been tested for, any family history of hidradenitis suppurative as up to 40% may have affected family members. Ask about general hygiene, regular shaving of affected areas, use of deodorant, any use of special washing agents. Ask for the presence of current symptoms such as fever, malaise, pain in affected areas that could signify the presence of an abscess that requires drainage.
iv. I would then examine the patient; check all sites affected by boils, check to see if the patient has boils that require incision and drainage, look for sinuses, take a pus swab of any discharging areas.
v. I would then devise a management plan.

- Lifestyle modification—lose weight (obesity is a risk factor), stop smoking, avoid irritating affected areas by shaving or use of perfume or perfumed deodorants, test for diabetes mellitus (recurrent boils may also be the first presentation of diabetes mellitus), optimize or maintain hygiene.

- Conservative—consider a course of antibiotics if the patient appears to have infected boils.
- Surgical—consider formal incision and drainage under local anesthesia or general anesthesia if the patient has abscesses that require drainage. Wide areas affected may require a skin graft, so in these instances, I would refer the patient to see a plastic surgeon.
- Referral to dermatology—various treatments offered such as contraceptive pill antiseptic washes, long-term antibiotics, and anti-inflammatories.

A follow-up question might be: What is the aetiology of hidradenitis suppurative?

- The underlying cause is thought to be occlusion of hair follicles with secondary involvement of the apocrine sweat glands leading to acute or chronic inflammation and destruction of these glands. Superadded infection leads to the formation of boils and abscesses.
- A second follow-up question might be: What are the risk factors for hidradenitis suppurative? Age (more common in adolescents and younger adults), gender (more common in females), family history, obesity and tobacco smoking.

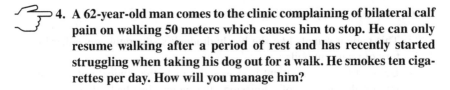 **4. A 62-year-old man comes to the clinic complaining of bilateral calf pain on walking 50 meters which causes him to stop. He can only resume walking after a period of rest and has recently started struggling when taking his dog out for a walk. He smokes ten cigarettes per day. How will you manage him?**

Example of how to approach this answer:

i. From the description, it would appear that the patient might have intermittent claudication although other differentials include osteoarthritis, spinal stenosis or lumbar nerve root entrapment.

ii. Before I bring the patient into the clinic room, I would check to see if there are any hematological or radiological results available and if the patient has previously been seen in outpatients or in A&E with this problem. A detailed history is crucial as this will usually help identify the underlying diagnosis.

iii. Next, I would bring the patient to clinic and take a detailed history:
   - Onset of symptoms.
   - Nature of the pain—cramping, tightening or tingling and location—calves, thighs, buttocks.
   - Is it unilateral or bilateral.
   - Is the pain felt at rest, while sitting down or after a certain distance of walking. Occasionally, mild claudication may be felt only when asking uphill or quickly.

- Any numbness, tingling, shooting pain.
- Any history of trauma or back pain.
- Impact of symptoms on activities of daily living and general functional status.
- PMHx—any history of smoking (amount/duration), ischemia, heart disease, diabetes mellitus, osteoarthritis, neurological disease.
- PSHx—any relevant surgical history.
- Drug history—use of aspirin, statins, beta-blockers.

iv. Next, I would examine the patient, focusing on the cardiovascular system and clinical signs to establish the site of peripheral vascular disease:

a. Calculate the body mass index (BMI), check blood pressure, test urine for glucose and assess hands for nicotine staining.
b. Assess all peripheral and central pulses, noting any arrhythmias such as atrial fibrillation.
c. Palpate the abdomen for aortic aneurysms.
d. Listen to the carotids for bruits.
e. Examine the lower limbs as follows:

- Inspection—any cyanosis or hyperemic appearance, presence of hair, presence of ulcers or sores.
- Palpation—temperature, pulses (start from proximal and proceed to distal), compare the pulses of each limb at a time: femoral, popliteal, dorsalis pedis, posterior tibial. Carry out Buerger's test: elevate the legs to at least 45 degrees, and then, with the patient sitting on the edge of the couch, dangle the feet down. Pallor on elevation and abnormal rubor or hyperemia on dependency is an important sign which indicates critical ischemia.
- Hand-held Doppler—auscultation with hand-held Doppler will establish arterial flow waveform and facilitate measurement of the ankle-brachial pressure index (ABPI). The ABPI measures the ratio of systolic blood pressure at the ankle to that in the arm and is an index of vessel competency. A value of 1 is normal.
- An ABPI of less than 0.5 suggests serving arterial disease and an ABPI of less than 0.3 is associated with critical ischemia.

v. Once a diagnosis of intermittent claudication is deemed as the main working diagnosis, I would devise a plan of management which will include additional investigations.

- Bloods tests—Full Blood Count to assess for anemia and polycythemia, biochemical profile to assess for diabetes and renal impairment, fasting lipid profile.
- I would arrange for the patient to have a color-flow duplex ultrasound that allows the visualization and hemodynamic assessment of the arteries. I would consider a CT angiogram if surgical or radiological intervention is likely to be required.

- I would spend a great deal of time counseling the patient about risk factor modification including smoking cessation, good diabetic control and optimization of blood pressure if indicated
- If available, I would refer the patient to a supervised exercise program. This may involve two hours of supervised exercise a week for a three-month period and advises people to exercise to the point of maximum pain to encourage the formation of collaterals.
- The patient may go on to definitively need angioplasty or bypass surgery.
- The national Institute for Health and Care Excellence (NICE) recommends prescribing naftidrofuryl oxalate if supervised exercise has not led to a satisfactory improvement, and the person prefers not to be referred for consideration of angioplasty or bypass surgery.

 5. A 61-year-old man is referred to the clinic with a painful lump in the right groin. The lump usually disappears when he lies flat. He has a pacemaker in situ and no other medical history. How will you manage him?

Example of how to approach this answer:

- From the information provided, the patient might have a symptomatic inguinal hernia. However, other differentials for a groin lump are lymphadenopathy, lump arising from skin or subcutaneous infection or a lump of vascular etiology such as saphena varix or iliac/femoral pseudo-aneurysm.
- Before I bring the patient into the clinic room, I would like to check if the patient has had previous presentations to the clinic or to A&E with this lump or if there are any results available such as ultrasound or CT imaging.
- I would then bring the patient in and take a detailed history to ascertain the following:

  - When the lump was first noticed.
  - How the lump was first noticed—because of associated symptoms or incidentally.
  - Whether the lump is increasing or decreasing in size if it is permanently visible or disappears.
  - Any previous groin surgery, any history of vascular disease, any other relevant past medical history—it is mentioned that the patient has a pacemaker which is going to be relevant in the operative management.
  - Patient's occupation and general functional status.

- I would then examine the patient: examine the abdomen and then the groin with the patient standing and lying down. If I can move the skin over the lump, then it is not within the skin layer. If it has a cough impulse, it is likely to be a hernia. If it is compressible or pulsator/expansile then it is likely to be of vascular origin.

  - For any lump, I consider the following aide memoir to cover all aspects of the description of the lump: 4 Ss, 4 Cs, 4 Ts:

- Size, size, shape, surface
- Color, contour, consistency, compressibility
- Tenderness, temperature, tethering, transillumenance

- You may be told at this stage that this is an inguinal hernia and asked follow-up questions:

  1. What is the definition of a hernia?

     - Protrusion of a viscus and its lining through a defect in its containing cavity into an abnormal position

  2. How do you differentiate an inguinal from a femoral hernia?

     - Broadly speaking, an inguinal hernia presents with a lump above and medial to the pubic tubercle, while a femoral hernia presents with a lump below and lateral to the pubic tubercle. Inguinal hernias are the most common type of groin hernias.

  3. What are the boundaries of the inguinal canal?

     - This is an intramuscular canal in the groin which is bounded anteriorly by the external oblique aponeurosis and internal oblique in the lateral 1/3, posterior by the transversalis fascia and conjoint tendon medially, its floor is formed by the inguinal ligament and its roof by the arching fibers of internal oblique.

  4. Would you offer this patient surgery? Is the presence of a pacemaker relevant?

     - This patient has a symptomatic inguinal hernia and is, therefore, a candidate for operative repair. For a unilateral, symptomatic inguinal hernia, the National Institute for Health and Care Excellence (NICE) recommends open tension-free repair using mesh. The most widely available technique is the Lichtenstein mesh repair. The presence of a pacemaker is important because it will determine the type of energy device that can be used at the time of surgery. In patients with pacemakers, avoid using diathermy if at all possible to avoid interference of the electrical current with the function of the pacemaker. If needed, then use bipolar diathermy to minimize current flow through the body.

3 Clinical Management Station

ABOUT THIS STATION

The clinical management station differs from the clinical station in that the emphasis here is on your capacity to use your management skills to solve clinical problems. It is designed to assess whether you can think beyond the clinical dilemma to other aspects of care, such as the availability of personnel and resources to assist you in managing the case. Like the clinical scenario, you will be given a clinical management scenario to read and prepare for. You will be provided with a pen and paper to take notes. After the preparation time, you will enter the station, and you will be asked to discuss your approach to managing the case. The interviewers are looking to see that you can appropriately delegate to junior colleagues and are not afraid to contact the consultant. In your answers, you should demonstrate that you neither shun responsibility nor attempt to take on everything at once. The scores will be based on parameters including situational awareness, judgment, setting priorities, managing the team, willingness to accept responsibility and involvement of other colleagues.

HOW TO TACKLE THIS STATION

1. Carefully read through the case provided and make sure that you have understood all of the information provided.
2. You can make notes to help you structure your answer, which should probably be in the form of bullet points. You must not spend too much time fussing over the notes as this could potentially reduce your preparation time.
3. Have a system of answering the question to apply this to any other clinical management situation that you encounter. In your answer, you should consider; the key issues in the case, if case prioritization is required, other members of the healthcare team that are available, what can be delegated and what instructions would you give to other team members.
4. You may wish to take the following steps when faced with a clinical management scenario:

   a. **Dilemma**—what is the clinical management dilemma?
   b. **Organize self**—what can I do?
   c. **Organize others**—who else is available and what can they do?
   d. **Manage situation**—how will we now manage the situation?
   e. **Escalate and communicate**—who else needs to be informed of the plans?
   f. **Draw everything together and summarize**—summarize the actions taken.

DOI: 10.1201/9781003221739-3

Following are examples of ten clinical management scenarios with a proposed answer. Each example will take you through how to deliver the answer and suggested further reading which is relevant to the topic.

CLINICAL MANAGEMENT SCENARIOS

 1. **You are the surgical registrar and your consultant has an after-noon elective list. You are in the admissions lounge consenting the two patients on the list; one is listed for laparoscopic chole-cystectomy and the other for reversal of loop ileostomy. As you begin consenting, you get a call from your SHO about an unwell patient on the ward who is four days post laparoscopic high anterior resection. The patient has taken a turn for the worst, and she is concerned about him. What will you do?**

   a. The issue here is that I have a sick patient on the ward that needs an urgent senior review, but at the same time, I have a list that is about to start.

   b. I would inform the anesthetist and theater staff that I have to attend an emergency on the ward and to not send for any of the patients just yet.

   c. I would then contact my consultant, explain the situation and check if he/she is able to come in and take over the consenting and starting of the list.

   d. I would inform the admissions' unit staff and the patients about the potential delay with the list's starting time.

   e. Once the consultant confirms that he/she is on their way in to start the list and the estimated time of arrival, I will update the theater team, admissions' lounge nurses and patient.

   f. I would ask the SHO to go to the theater and assist the consultant, while I go and review the unwell patient with the HO/FY1.

   g. Once I get to the ward, I would manage the patient in concordance with the principles of CCrISP.

   h. Depending on the condition of the patient, I may then be able to rejoin the elective list, or I may have to prepare the unwell patient for definitive care, which may include emergency surgery.

   i. Either way, I will ensure that my consultant is kept updated with the events.

 2. **You are the on-call registrar who has just started a night shift. Immediately after the night handover, you get a call from the ward sister about a patient who had an extended right hemicolectomy three days ago who has become pyrexic and tachycardia and has excruciating abdominal pain. At the same time, your SHO get a call from the A&E nurse in charge about two surgical patients who have been waiting for almost 3.5 hours in A&E; one has a buttock abscess**

and the other is deeply jaundiced. **The SHO has been told that both have a Medical Early Warning Score (MEWS) score of 1. How would you manage this scenario?**

a. The issue here is that three patients need to be seen urgently, but the sickest of them is the inpatient on the ward who has become acutely unwell.

b. The sickest of the three patients, the patient on the ward, is the first to require a senior review.

c. I would send the SHO to A&E to review the two patients that are waiting. I would give the SHO clear advice about the worrying features to look out for that need to be escalated to me right away, e.g. if the patient with the buttock abscess has features suggestive of necrotizing fasciitis and if the jaundiced patient might be cholangitic.

d. I would go to the ward to assess the unwell patient and take the on-call HO/FY1 to review the patient with me.

e. Once on the ward, I would manage the patient according to the principles of CCrISP:

    i. ABCDE ensuring O_2, intravenous access, intravenous fluids, Sepsis 6 bundle initiated

    ii. History—symptoms, op notes, team the patient is under, diagnosis and treatment so far, comorbid conditions and other relevant information such as ceiling of care, resuscitation status and P-POSSUM score

    iii. Examination

    iv. Review of charts and results

    v. Management plan as guided by the findings and the HO/FY1 to assist with requesting tests or further investigations

    vi. Relay the management plan to the patient and nursing staff and/or on-call consultant depending on the state of the patient

f. Catch up with SHO and review the two patients in A&E.

3. **You are the ST3 on the firm and your consultant asked you to book an emergency laparoscopic cholecystectomy to do first thing the following morning. You make the relevant arrangements, and you turn up to the emergency theater the next morning to find the CEPOD coordinator doesn't have the booking form and that two other consultants have cases to do. Your consultant is on her way, but her phone is off. What do you do?**

a. The key issues here are that:

    • My case is not on the CEPOD list even though I booked it.

    • My consultant expects to start with this case but cannot be contacted.

    • Other consultants want to start their cases ahead of the emergency cholecystectomy.

- I would address this dilemma as follows:
- Seek information

  - What are the cases that the other consultants want to do and are they more urgent than the emergency laparoscopic cholecystectomy?
  - How unwell are those patients by comparison?
  - Explore what happened to my booking form and if a new one needs to be filled out, ask the SHO to do it right away to avoid delays. I may need to fill in an incident form if this is a recurring theme, but I can deal with this later.

- Patient safety/care

  - We need to do what is best for the patients and prioritize the emergencies. The Royal College of Surgeons document on good surgical practice advocates that patients are prioritized and treated according to their clinical need.
  - I would reassess my patient to check how he/she is today and whether the other two emergencies now take priority.

- Initiative and support

  - Once I have reassessed my patient, I would set up a meeting with the other consultant surgeons and the on-call anesthetist and theater coordinator to prioritize the cases. I would try to contact my consultant once again.
  - Ultimately, we all want the best care for our patients without any conflict. Therefore, it is important that we have an open dialogue, negotiate and reach a unanimous decision about the order of cases.
  - I would explore the possibility of doing our case in another theater too if other lists have had cancellations—this can be discussed with the theater co-ordinator.
  - I would also keep my patients and ward staff updated on the estimated time of surgery.

4. **You are the ST3 and you're scrubbed in with the consultant to do an open abdominal aortic aneurysm (AAA) repair. You have previously assisted with one open AAA repair. Your consultant places the clamp on the infra-renal aorta. Soon after this, your consultant collapses with chest pain. What would you do?**

  - The issues are twofold:

    - We have an anesthetized patient on the table with an open abdomen who is in the middle of a major operation that I am not competent at doing alone.
    - The lead Surgeon who is my consultant has become acutely unwell and is now an emergency.

- I would ask the theater staff to put out a cardiac arrest call and for my consultant to be taken into the anesthetic room for cardiopulmonary resuscitation to begin. The whole cardiac arrest team will arrive within minutes to continue managing him.
- The patient on the table is now my responsibility, and since the aortic clamp has been positioned, we have a maximum of four hours to complete the operation so that the clamp can be removed.
- I need to remain scrubbed, but I will ask the SHO or theater staff to contact the on-call consultant and ask them to come to the theater.
- If the on-call consultant is not available, or is available but not able to perform an emergency open AAA repair, we will need to contact another consultant on-site who may have the expertise.
- If not, we will need to contact the nearest vascular unit and ask for their on-call vascular consultant to come out to our hospital.
- In the meantime, we could ask for assistance from a transplant surgeon or plastic surgeon who would have experience in vascular surgery.
- This is the type of situation that should be discussed in the weekly departmental meeting and clinical governance meetings to highlight any areas for improvement.
- I would fill out an incident form.

 5. **You are the on-call surgical registrar and you have been fast-bleeped to Resus. You arrive with the on-call surgical SHO. There are two patients in Resus: Patient 1 is day one post laparoscopic cholecystectomy and has a MEWS score of 8. Patient 2 is actively hemorrhaging from his torso and right leg after falling through a shattered glass window on the second floor. How do you proceed?**

- The issue here is that both patients are seriously unwell and require urgent surgical attention, but I can only see one at a time.
- I will review the hemorrhaging trauma patient and delegate the assessment of the post laparoscopic cholecystectomy patient to the SHO.
- I would immediately put out a trauma call to assemble the full trauma team to manage this multiply-injured patient.
- I would lead the trauma call as per the ATLS protocol, ensuring that the patient has airway maintenance with restriction of the cervical spine motion, breathing and ventilation assessment, circulation and hemorrhage control, including the application of direct pressure to any actively bleeding points activating the major hemorrhage protocol. I would continue with the rest of the primary survey, addressing all life-threatening pathology first before moving on to the secondary survey.

- While the patient is being stabilized with the rest of the trauma team present, I will catch up with the SHO and review the returning post-operative patient and inform the on-call consultant as indicated.
- I would debrief with the SHO later on and use the opportunity to discuss the case and complete a work-based assessment.

6. **You have an elective list today with the consultant, but the consultant has just texted you to say that he will not be available for the next three hours. You have a theater list with four cases, and you can only independently do the first two. However, one of these patients has just had some food, and the other requires a check of her international normalized ratio (INR). What will you do?**

- The issue here is that my consultant is not available for part of the list and the list has four cases, but I can only do two independently. Ideally, I would have liked to start with these two but for patient-related factors, this cannot happen. Also, most importantly, I do not have consultant cover for half of the list.
- This list will almost certainly be delayed, and the order of the cases will need to be revised.
- First, I will try and get some information about the consultant's unavailability. Is he or she in a meeting on-site or off-site? How long will he or she be away for? Has he/she delegated another consultant to cover the list in his absence?
- At this stage, it is vitally important to keep everyone in the loop:

  - Inform the anesthetist, the theater staff, the admissions' lounge or ward nursing staff (depending on where the elective patients are) and the patients about the situation which is going to cause a delay in the start of the list and a change in the order of cases.

- Get the HO/FY1 to take an urgent sample for INR for the patient that needs this checked and to run it to the lab urgently.
- Keep the patient who has eaten NBM from this point onwards.
- Suppose my consultant is going to be away for three hours but will return after that. In that case, as long as there is another consultant covering the list, I can start the first case when the INR is back, and when the original responsible consultant arrives, we can resume with the second case.
- If the consultant is going to be away for the whole list, provided he or she has delegated another consultant to cover the list, I can start the first case when the INR is back and get the delegated consultant to help me from the second case onward.
- If the consultant is unavailable and has not delegated another consultant, then I will need to find out if he or she would be happy for the on-call consultant to supervise me.
- If I cannot get hold of my consultant, and cannot determine his or her wishes, and there is no delegated consultant to be in charge of

the list, then I will have to cancel all of the cases. An incident form will need to be completed.

- Generally speaking, it is important to try as far as possible not to cancel cases on the day since it inconveniences patients, wastes resources and bears financial penalties for the Trust. However, a list should not proceed without consultant cover.
- If cases are canceled, I will ensure that the waiting-list coordinator is informed so that they can reschedule the patients.
- I will ensure that the situation is fully documented.

7. **You are the ST3 about to start your ward round this morning. You have foundation year 1 and year 2 doctors on the ward duties with you. As you take the handover from the night team about your patients, you find out that your anterior resection patient who is four days post-op is tachycardic and has a temperature of 39 degrees Celsius. Another one of your ward patients is now complaining of a swollen leg and has become hypoxic. The Foundation year 1 doctor comes to the ward smelling of alcohol. You have a ward-round to do and then a teaching theater list arranged by your consultant. What would you do?**

- The key issues here are that I have two unwell patients on the ward that need a senior review, an unsafe HO/FY1 as, a ward-round to do and a list in the afternoon to prepare for.
- I will plan to begin the ward-round by reviewing the post-op patient who may have an anastomotic leak and get the FY2 to review the second patient who may have a DVT and PE and report back to make. I will give the FY2 clear advice about resuscitation of the patient (ensuring airway is secure, optimizing oxygenation, getting intravenous access, getting appropriate investigations such as bloods, ABG, CXR, ECG) and report back to me as soon as he/she has seen the patient.
- The HO/FY1 who smells of alcohol is unsafe and lacks insight and must therefore leave the clinical area. This is a serious matter relating to conduct and I will inform my consultant about it and arrange a meeting at the earliest opportunity with the FY1 and the consultant. This matter will need to be escalated to his or her Educational Supervisor. I will ensure that the FY1 goes home safely.
- It is important to keep everyone in the loop, so prior to reviewing the two unwell patients:

  - Inform the responsible consultant about the emergencies on the ward, which will delay the ward-round and possibly the list.
  - Inform the consultant about the HO/FY1 that you've had to send home.
  - It may be prudent to postpone the rest of the ward-round to do between cases because by then I will have the FY2 to go around with me and we can get through the ward-round more quickly.

- Inform the anesthetist, theater staff and theater coordinator that the list may be delayed a little and to not send for any of the patients until I get back to them.

- Review the anterior resection patient and resuscitate and manage according to the principles of CCrISP.
- Catch up with the FY2 and then resume the list when appropriate to do so.
- In the meantime, I may need to arrange for another junior to assist the consultant with the list.

8. **You are about to start a laparoscopic appendicectomy and are called by the intensive treatment unit about a patient with generalized peritonitis who they suspect may have a perforated peptic ulcer. What would you do?**

- The key issues here are that I am about to start an operation, but the intensive treatment unit (ITU) have a peritonitic patient that needs an urgent senior surgical review.
- First, I need to find out if the appendicectomy case is anesthetized. If so, we will need to proceed with the operation. In this instance, I will have to call the on-call consultant to take over from me.
- If the patient is awake but stable:

  - Inform the anesthetist and theater staff about the emergency on ITU that may require a laparotomy.
  - Since the appendicectomy patient is stable, I will ask the anaesthetist not to anaesthetize the patient until I get in contact with him.
  - I will explain the situation to the patient and apologize to them.

- I will make my way to ITU, and on the way, get the HO/FY1 or SHO to join me.
- Review the unwell patient on ITU and manage as per the principles of CCrISP.
- If the patient requires a laparotomy, he or she may need to be prioritized ahead of the appendicectomy. If the patient requires further imaging, then delegate to the surgical SHO and ITU team to arrange for the scans. Depending on how long this is likely to take, and if the consultant on call is available, it may be possible to clear the appendicectomy case while the ITU patient is being resuscitated and scanned.
- I will need to stay in close communication with my consultant, the CEPOD team and ITU.

9. **You are the ST3 on call for general surgery, and you have an SHO and FY1. There is no vascular service in your hospital. A trauma call has been put out following a major collision between two cars.**

The patients in one car are en route: a man with an open fracture and acute leg ischemia, a woman who is 32 weeks pregnant and has abdominal pain, a 10-year-old boy who is shocked and complaining of RUQ pain who has his father with him.

- The situation is that this is a level 1 major incident with three casualties including an obstetrics and pediatrics emergency.
- Given that there were two cars involved, there is likely to be more injured patients en route.
- A trauma call has been put out.
- I will also put out an obstetrics emergency call and a pediatric emergency call.
- I will request at this point that the patients from the second car get diverted to another unit and will get our site manager and A&E nurse in charge involved in this.
- While we are waiting for the patients to arrive, I will take the lead and divide the team up as follows:

  - A&E SpR and orthopedic SpR to lead the management of the man with open fracture and limb ischemia as the limb ischaemia is likely to be secondary to complications from the open fracture.
  - Obstetrics SpR to lead management of pregnant woman.
  - I will lead the management of the shocked child with the paediatric SpR.

- Have the porters on stand-by to run blood off and retrieve blood from the blood bank.
- Manage each of the cases as per the ATLS protocol, ensuring that all of the juniors are involved and utilized appropriately.
- I will try as far as possible to communicate with the other two leads of the two cases as they may still have general surgical or vascular emergencies.
- If a child is peritonitic, then:

  - Inform the anesthetist on call who will be in A&E.
  - Inform my consultant and ask him/her to come in.
  - Make arrangements for theater.
  - Speak to the anaesthetist oncall.
  - SHO to book the case and bleep theater coordinator.
  - Speak to the father of the child if now stable and get his consent for surgery for the child.
  - If the father is unwell and or not the one with parental responsibility, then manage the child in his/her best interests and continue with arrangements for theater.

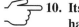 10. **Its 7:30 on the morning of your consultant's all-day list. You have a reversal of ileostomy, a sigmoid colectomy and an anterior**

resection on your list. **Your consultant has told you he wants you to assist him as he intends to take you through the operations and expects you to be able to do them at least in part by the end of your attachment with him and he feels it is appropriate for your level to be with him. He told you the day before to consent everyone (you can) and get the first patient on the table by 8:30 when he will be in to join you but is in a meeting and unavailable till then.**

Next to your theaters, one of the staff grades has a minor ops list with two hernias, a lap chole and a lipoma excision.

The staff grade takes you aside and tells you he thinks it would be best if you swapped lists. Laparoscopic cholecystectomies and hernias are better for you, and he would be better learning the more complicated things which are currently above your level. You have consented all your patients at this point. He has not consented to any of his. The anaesthetists are not aware of his intentions.

How do you manage this situation?

Clearly, this is a difficult situation for several reasons.

Patient safety issues

- I know my patients and I have fully prepared them for theater.
- I know their background, and this is relevant given that they are having major operations.
- The staff grade does not know these patients.
- Therefore, from a safety point of view, I am best placed to be doing these operations.

Communication and organizational issues

- The anesthetists and theater staff have no knowledge of this and my anaesthetist, theater staff, consultant and patients expect me to be doing the list.
- Last-minute changes to lists are considered as unsafe behaviors, which have been implicated in a report published on the Royal College of Surgeons (RCS) website (commissioning the conditions for safer surgery—2014) as one of the main causes of never events.

Training issues

- My consultant wants me to learn these operations and wants to teach me.
- Giving up my list will not only negatively impact upon my training, it will also antagonize my consultant.

I will politely refuse using the reasons mentioned earlier.

PRIORITIZATION AND COMMUNICATION

You may be given a list of patients as part of the clinical management station or the communication station to speak to your consultant about. Typically, this will be a list of about 10–15 patients, and for each patient, there will be a few sentences describing the clinical situation. You will then be asked to pick up the telephone and talk to the consultant about them over a very short phone call. You consultant may even signpost at the start that he or she only has two minutes to talk. The key challenge with this station is having to prioritize which patients to talk to the consultant about. There will not be time to talk about every patient. Equally, the consultant may not want to hear about the status of every single patient on your list, e.g. the one with a thrombosed hemorrhoid who is going home with conservative management. Having a system to establishing how to start the conversation is crucial.

HOW TO TACKLE THIS STATION

You will be provided with a pen and paper to make notes. You may find it useful to divide the page up into four quadrants according to clinical priority/need and label the quadrants (1 to 4, 1 denoting highest and 4 lowest clinical priority) as follows:

- Quadrant 1—needs surgery
- Quadrant 2—unwell patients
- Quadrant 3—needs transfer
- Quadrant 4—stable or going home

Imagine the following is your A4 sheet of notepaper

1. *Needs surgery*	2. *Unwell patients*
3. *Needs transfer*	4. *Stable or going home*

i. As you read through the list of patients, place the patients in the appropriate quadrants.
ii. Once you start speaking to the consultant, start with quadrant 1 and work your way around to quadrant 4. By doing this, you will find that you have spoken to your consultant about the patients in order of clinical priority, from most to least.
iii. You will be challenged at some point, possibly with an incorrect suggestion so it's important to think and not to agree immediately.
iv. Signpost early that you have patients to discuss about what you think is the priority and just go through as many as you can until the bell rings.
v. For on-call scenarios: divide patients up into the following quadrants:

- **Quadrant 1—for surgery**
- **Quadrant 2—unwell**
- **Quadrant 3—for transfer**
- **Quadrant 4—stable or going home**

vi. For clinic scenarios: divide patients up into the following quadrants:

- **Quadrant 1—admit**
- **Quadrant 2—urgent investigations**
- **Quadrant 3—routine follow-up/waiting list**
- **Quadrant 4—discharge**

PRIORITIZATION SCENARIOS

1. You are the ST3 doing a general clinic. List of the following patients in clinic to discuss with the consultant on the phone.

a. 50M presenting 1 week after inguinal hernia repair with a tender groin lump
b. 65F presenting with an incisional hernia. Speaks no English and there are no notes
c. 18F presenting with abdominal pain and having active fresh rectal bleeding
d. 75M presenting with an anal mass of unclear etiology. The patient is well and not clinically obstructed.
e. 26F presenting with symptomatic hemorrhoids
f. 45M presenting with a symptomatic paraumbilical hernia with no features of acute incarceration of the hernia or bowel obstruction

- Quadrant 1: Admit: Patients a, c
- Quadrant 2: Urgent investigations: Patient d
- Quadrant 3: Routine follow-up/waiting list: Patients b, e, f
- Quadrant 4: Discharge: None

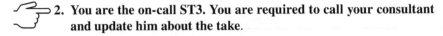**2. You are the on-call ST3. You are required to call your consultant and update him about the take**.

a. A female patient with gallstones complaining of acute right upper quadrant pain. Normal liver function tests and amylase. CRP 10.

b. A renal dialysis male patient whose arterio-venous fistula is not working.

c. A 10-year-old girl with mild right iliac fossa pain and normal blood results. She recently had a throat infection.

d. A female patient with Crohn's disease with a seton in situ following previous drainage of perianal abscess. She now has a large perianal abscess and is septic.

e. A 65-year-old man with right iliac fossa pain and localized peritonitis.

f. A patient who had a laparoscopic cholecystectomy earlier in the day and is now tachycardic and hypotensive and is deteriorating in spite of resuscitation.

g. A patient with peripheral vascular disease who has presented with a gangrenous left big toe.

h. A medical patient with known ulcerative colitis who has a dilated colon on AXR and is septic.

i. A 19-year-old man with acute left testicular pain.

j. A patient who had an open hysterectomy 2 days earlier who now has bowel visible through the wound, according to the obstetrics and gynecology Registrar.

- Quadrant 1: For surgery: Patients d, f, h, i, j
- Quadrant 2: Unwell: Patients e (needs urgent CTAP)
- Quadrant 3: For transfer: Patients b, g (to a vascular unit)
- Quadrant 4: For observation: Patients a, c

3. **You are the on-call ST3. You are required to call your consultant and update him about the take.**

a. 90F with a 10-hour history acute limb ischaemia on a background of atrial fibrillation.

b. 35M who is 7 days post-paraumbilical hernia repair and now has a minor wound infection with no underlying collection.

c. 65M who is 5 days post-laparoscopic anterior resection; he has absolute constipation and is complaining of worsening abdominal pain. His CRP is rising.

d. 10F with a good history of appendicitis.

e. 30F presenting with a one day history of right iliac fossa pain and has normal bloods.

f. 50M presenting with left iliac fossa pain and has raised inflammatory markers.

g. 45F with gallstone pancreatitis and a Glasgow score of 3.

- Quadrant 1: For surgery: Patients a (for embolectomy if local vascular services are available), d

- Quadrant 2: Unwell: Patients c, f, g
- Quadrant 3: For transfer: Patient a if local vascular services are not available
- Quadrant 4: For observation: Patients b, e

4 Academic Station

This station is often the most feared when it comes to interview preparation. Candidates will be provided with an abstract to read and subsequently be asked to present an opinion and answer questions relating to research. Before you begin to critically appraise research, it is important to understand the following concepts:

- Evidence-based medicine
- Levels of evidence
- Study design—meta-analysis; randomized control trials; observational studies
- Study reporting guidelines
- Statistics

EVIDENCE-BASED MEDICINE

This is defined as "the conscious, explicit and judicious use of current best evidence in making decisions about the care of individual patients". The practice of evidence-based medicine (EBM) means integrating individual clinical expertise with the best available clinical evidence from systematic research.

EBM takes into account the following:

- Best research evidence
- Clinical expertise and available resources
- Patients' values and preferences

Steps involved in EBM:

1. Main question
2. Construct a clinical question from the main question that needs to be answered
3. For treatment use; PICO—Population Intervention Comparison Outcome
4. Conduct research
5. Appraise evidence
6. Integrate evidence into practice to find a solution
7. Evaluate results

Why use clinical expertise in EBM?

A study or paper may be the best available regarding a particular topic; however, it may not be relevant to a particular patient. Patients often have comorbidities that may influence clinical decision making and may not be addressed fully in the papers being studied.

DOI: 10.1201/9781003221739-4

LEVELS OF EVIDENCE

An important aspect of evidence-based medicine is the hierarchical system of categorizing evidence, from the strongest type of evidence as level 1 to the weakest type of evidence, level 5.

1a. Systematic review or meta-analysis of randomized control trials (RCT)
1b. At least one RCT
2a. At least one well-designed control study without randomization
2b. One quasi-experimental study, e.g., cohort study
3. Nonexperimental descriptive studies, e.g., comparative, correlation, case-control and case series
4. Expert committee report/opinions +– clinical experience
5. Individual experience such as case report

STUDY DESIGNS

SYSTEMATIC REVIEW

- A summary of the high-quality existing research on the topic
- This type of evidence is the highest level of evidence
- There is a standardized method for conducting systematic reviews
- All available research, including published non-English work is used
- Relevant studies are combined using meta-analysis
- The best-known collection of systematic reviews is the Cochrane collaboration

META-ANALYSIS

- Involves combining results from several studies into a standardized measure to produce stronger evidence. Note that the results will only be as good as the material used. A good meta-analysis on flawed research produces flawed results. There is no limit on the number of studies that can be included in the meta-analysis.

RANDOMIZED CONTROL TRIALS

These are studies whereby interventions are randomly allocated to patients to avoid bias. There are two groups: placebo groups that are not being treated (controls) and intervention groups (treated). Interventions are randomly allocated to each group.

The types of control groups may be:

- Treatment vs no treatment
- Treatment vs placebo (looks like treatment but is not)
- Test treatment vs another type of treatment (to prove that one is superior to the other)

- Dose–response treatment (subjects randomly allocated to different doses)
- Cross-over—treatment is switched between the two groups after a period of time

These types of studies may be:

- *Open*—the researcher and the participants know groups and treatments. Very difficult to remove bias
- *Blind*

  - Single-blind—researcher knows, but the participant does not know (blind)—researcher bias
  - Double-blind—neither researcher nor participant knows (both blind)—little bias
  - Triple blind—neither researcher, participant or person administering treatment know—very little bias

OBSERVATIONAL STUDY

- Cohort—a retrospective type of study that analyses "risk factors." A cohort is a group of individuals who share common characteristics or experiences within a defined period. This type of study follows a group of individuals who share a common characteristic over a period of time and establishes those afflicted by the disease. For example, all smokers followed up over 40 years to see who gets lung cancer.
- Case-control—a retrospective type of study. In a case-control study, people with a disease (the cases) are compared to those who do not have the disease (the controls). Further data are then collected from the groups to determine if other characteristics are also different between the two groups.
- Cross-sectional—this type of study follows participants up over a period of time once they have had an intervention. They were usually used to look at the possible effects of treatment on patients.

STUDY REPORTING GUIDELINES

Reporting guidelines contain a checklist of baseline points and guidance that are required when reporting research. They help to improve the reliability of published research by promoting clear reporting of methods and results. There are different guidelines for different study designs. The most frequently encountered guidelines for common study designs are:

- CONSORT (Consolidated Standards of Reporting Trials) guidelines for randomized controlled trials
- PRISMA (Preferred Reporting Items for Systematic Reviews and Meta-Analyses) guidelines for systematic reviews
- STROBE (Strengthening the Reporting of Observational Studies in Epidemiology) guidelines for observational studies

Important statistical and research concepts to study the definitions for:

- Type 1 error vs Type 2 error
- Odds ratio; relative risk; confidence interval
- Study power and sample size
- Mode; median; mean
- Standard error; standard deviation
- Number to treat vs odds ratio
- Negative predictive value (NPV) vs positive predictive value
- Funnel plot; Kaplan Meier; histogram; Box–Whisker; Forrest plots
- T-test, Mann–Whitney, ANOVA, logistic regression
- Allocation concealment and blinding
- Impact factor
- Publication bias
- Clinical and methodological heterogenicity
- Intention to treat vs per-protocol analysis
- Internal and external validity
- Trial design: superiority; equivalence; non-inferiority

 CRITICAL APPRAISAL OF RESEARCH

Critical appraisal is the systematic process by which clinicians review and analyze the available evidence to determine its significance and relevance to clinical practice. It enables clinicians to draw appropriate conclusions about the usefulness and validity of the published evidence and forms the cornerstone of surgical practice.
Targets of critical appraisal:

- Original quantitative research
- Reviews (systematic reviews and meta-analyses)
- Original qualitative research

Steps to follow:

1. Summarize the research

    - What journal was this study published in and when?
    - What type of study design, and what is the level of evidence according to the Oxford hierarchy?
    - What is the aim of the study?
    - Is the study retrospective or prospective (if observational)?
    - What is the follow-up duration?
    - What are the primary outcomes?
    - What is the sample size?
    - What is the main result(s), and is this statistically significant?
    - What were the main conclusions drawn?

2. Identify and comment on the relevant strengths and weaknesses of the study based on what you have read. The following factors will need to be considered:

- Type of journal and impact factor
- Institution – Academic? Non-western study?
- Relevance/importance of the topic
- Level of evidence
- A single or multicentre study
- Sample size
- Potential confounding factors (were these accounted for?)
- Inclusion and exclusion criteria
- Limitation of bias (selection criteria; open vs blind; intention to treat vs per-protocol analysis)
- Clinical and methodological heterogenicity
- Were the study guidelines followed?
- Clinical outcomes

3. Apply the evidence to clinical practice. Before establishing whether the piece of research is useful to your practice, it is important to acknowledge to the interviewer that you will be required to read the paper in full, review the background and study design before making any application to clinical practice. The following questions will help guide your decision process:

- Has this research provided useful conclusions (accepted or rejected their hypothesis)?
- Does it apply to the population of patients that you are looking to treat?
- Do the benefits outweigh the risks of implementing said intervention or practice to your particular patient population?
- Is it feasible to implement this intervention or practice in your current setting?

On the day of the interview, you will be provided with an abstract or a short research article. The information provided in this chapter will enable you to systemically approach the critical appraisal of any article. You may find it useful to practice appraising and presenting research articles to colleagues ahead of the interview and remember to ask for feedback. Practice makes perfect!

5 Technical Skills Station

In this station, the applicant has 8–10 minutes to perform a technical task. This station aims to assess the candidate's teaching skills as well as their technical ability. During your preparation, practice the common procedures, as outlined in the Basic Surgical Skills course, to ensure that you gain fluency in the technical aspects. It can be quite daunting to teach the procedure while performing it in an interview setting; therefore, get into the habit of talking through the steps of the procedure out loud while practicing. It is also worth practicing performing these skills with junior members of your team and asking for their feedback on your teaching skills. Ask senior colleagues (registrars, consultants) for feedback on your technique and ask for feedback if appropriate.

The Pendleton method of feedback is commonly used throughout medicine and you may find it helpful in obtaining the feedback:

1. What do you think went well?
2. What I thought went well was . . .
3. Is there anything you would do differently?
4. What I might have done differently is . . .

It is important to have a structure for this station to ensure that all the necessary points are covered. Most teaching courses use a four-stage model to demonstrate how to teach procedures:

1. Perform the procedure as you would in real life
2. Repeat the procedure more slowly, while describing the steps
3. Repeat the procedure, and this time ask the trainee to describe the steps
4. Ask the trainee to perform the procedure

If you are asked in the interview how you would teach a skill, you may wish to refer to the four-step approach described earlier. For the interview, you may find it useful to describe out loud what you are performing as you go through it. This will serve as an aide-memoir to guide you through the procedure and demonstrate to the interviewer that you understand the steps involved.

The following is a framework for completing this station using the example of excision of a skin lesion. It incorporates the models we have discussed:

1. Introduction

   a. *Hello, my name is . . .*
   b. *Do you have any experience with this procedure?*

DOI: 10.1201/9781003221739-5

2. Set out the objectives

   a. *Today, we will go through the appropriate steps for this procedure includ-ing the instruments needed.*

3. Set out the teaching method

   a. *I will describe the steps of the procedure while I perform them.*

4. State the pre-operative preparation that will be conducted before the proce-dure is undertaken. For example:

   a. *We have gone through the World Health Organization surgical safety checklist.*
   b. *The surgical field has been cleaned with antiseptic skin solution and draped using an aseptic technique.*
   c. *We have infiltrated local anesthetic into the skin.*

5. List the appropriate instruments—you may have to pick these out of a set.

   a. *In this example: fine-toothed Gillie's forceps, a no. 15 blade, a needle holder, a non-absorbable monofilament suture on a cutting needed (3–0 nylon), toothed forceps and a marker pen.*

6. Describe the procedure as you perform it

   a. *I am marking out 3mm margins and drawing an ellipse which is three times longer than the width to enable skin closure without excess tension.*
   b. *I am using the toothed forceps to check that the skin is anesthetized.*
   c. *I am incising along with the markings while holding the scalpel like a pen (Figure A).*
   d. *I have joined the incision at one end.*
   e. *I am lifting one end of the lesion as I excise it with my scalpel (Figure B),*
   f. *I am marking the medial end of the specimen with a non-absorbable suture and I will note this on the request form as I send the specimen for histology.*
   g. *I am closing the skin using interrupted mattress sutures, starting at the ends and working toward the middle (Figure C).*

7. Reiterate the teaching model

   a. *On our next case together, I will ask you to describe the steps for me while I excise another skin lesion, and then, I will ask you to excise a skin lesion yourself.*

8. Feedback—using the Pendleton model

   a. *The interviewer is unlikely to answer any questions asked.*
   b. *Depending on the amount of time available, it may be worth just men-tioning during the interview that you would ask for feedback using the Pendleton model.*

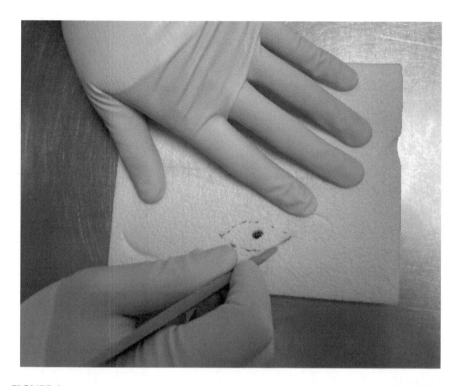

FIGURE A

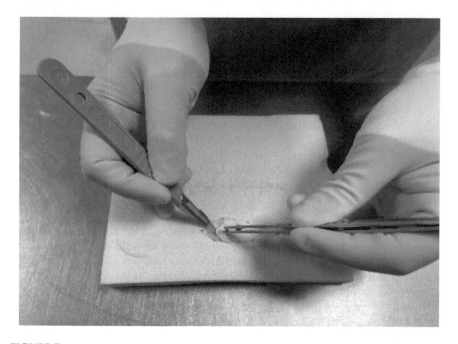

FIGURE B

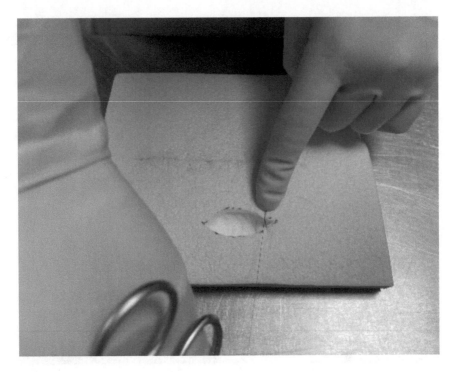

FIGURE C

9. Check that the learning objectives have been achieved
10. End with advice

   a. *Keep practicing these skills at home and attend a Basic Surgical Skills course if you are interested in this.*
   b. *Would you please send me a work-based assessment for this procedure?*

The following are two further examples of technical skills you may be asked to demonstrate:

Demonstrate and teach how to tie a surgeon's knot

Hello, my name is x. Today, we will go through how to tie a surgeon's knot. Do you have any experience with this procedure?

We will go through the steps for this procedure, including the instruments needed. I will describe the steps of the procedure while I perform them. We have gone through the WHO checklist already. This skin has been prepped and draped using an aseptic technique. We have infiltrated local anesthetic into the skin. We will now use a braided suture on a cutting needle such as 2–0 Vicryl. We will hold this using needle holders and will also require toothed forceps and straight scissors.

I am using the toothed forceps to evert the skin edge and I am inserting the needle perpendicular to the skin edge. I am supinating my wrist to drive the needle through the skin edge (Figure D).

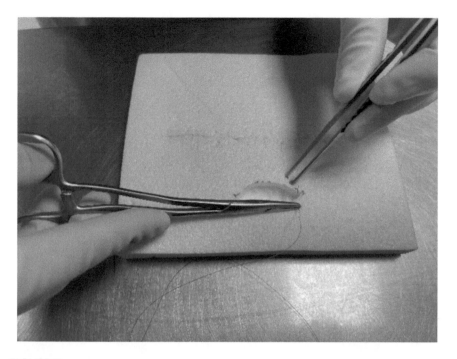

FIGURE D

I will now do this for the other side as well. To be careful with the needle, I will hold the end of the thread with the needle hanging between my thumb and ring fingers of my left hand. The other end of the suture goes vertically over my index and middle fingers of my left hand in the other direction, and I use my middle finger to tie the knot (Figure E).

At this stage, I will perform two loops instead of just one to tie a surgeon's knot. I will tighten the knot just enough to appose the skin edges. I will use my index finger to snug the knot down in the best position to one side of the skin incision. I will then use the straight scissors to cut off the excess suture leaving 5 mm behind. I will dispose of the needle in a sharps bin. This suture will need removal after 10 days.

On our next case together, I will ask you to describe the steps for me while I tie another surgeon's knot and then I will ask you to tie a surgeon's knot yourself.

Do you have any questions? Have we appropriately covered our objectives? Keep practicing tying knots at home and be sure to attend a Basic Surgical Skills course if you are interested in developing your skills further. Would you please send me a work-based assessment for this procedure?

If time permits, I would like to ask for feedback using the Pendleton method.

Demonstrate and teach how to perform a small bowel anastomosis

Good afternoon, my name is x. Today we will go through how to perform a small bowel anastomosis. Do you have any experience with this procedure?

We will go through the steps for this procedure and the equipment required. I will describe the steps of the procedure while I perform them. We have gone through the

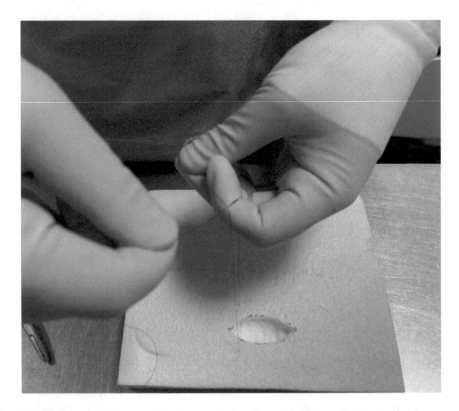

FIGURE E

WHO checklist already, and the surgical field has been prepped and draped using an aseptic technique. We will use non-toothed Debakey forceps to handle the bowel and an absorbable monofilament suture on a round-bodied needle such as 3–0 PDS. We will also need a needle holder, two hemostats and straight scissors.

We need to ensure that the bowel ends match. The strongest layer of the bowel wall is the submucosa, so we must include this in the anastomosis. There are several techniques for small bowel anastomosis. I will use the interrupted sutures technique. I will insert two stay sutures at the mesenteric and antimesenteric borders and place them in hemostats instead of tying them. I will ask you to hold the hemostats to provide me with traction on the bowel edges. I am passing my stitches vertically through the layers of the bowel wall, 3–4 mm from the edge and 3–4 mm apart. I am hand-tying my knots using surgeon's knots. I am inverting the bowel edges to bury the mucosa and ensuring appropriate tension throughout. When I have completed the anterior layer, I will turn the bowel over to suture the posterior wall by passing my stay suture under the bowel to the opposite side. I will then tie the stay sutures and cut them appropriately.

On our next case together, I will ask you to describe the steps for me while I perform another small bowel anastomosis, and then, I will ask you to perform the procedure yourself whilst I supervise.

Do you have any questions? Have we appropriately covered our objectives? Keep practicing these techniques at home and be sure to attend a Basic Surgical Skills course

if you are interested in developing your skills further. Would you please send me a work-based assessment for this procedure?
If time permits, I would like to ask for feedback using the Pendleton method.

The scenarios used in this station can vary from year to year and are usually taught on the Basic Surgical Skills course. It is worthwhile watching the Basic Surgical Skills Course DVD to help prepare for this station. The list below outlines additional examples of technical skills that may be assessed in this station. You may wish to prepare answers for them using the format outlined earlier and practice this with your contemporaries.

- Perform a vein patch/transverse arteriotomy
- Perform a femoral embolectomy
- Laparoscopically excise a circle
- Laparoscopically perform two interrupted sutures

6 Ethics Station

The Royal College of Surgeon's Good Surgical Practice guidance highlights key ethical and legal principles fundamental to everyday surgical practice. During the interview, you will be tested on your understanding of these concepts and your ability to implement them practically. Although there is no specific ethics station at present, you will be expected to identify ethical issues within clinical and clinical management scenarios and discuss how you would address the situation.

The four fundamental ethical principles:

- Beneficence—acting in the patient's best interest
- Nonmaleficence—doing no harm
- Justice—all patients must be treated equally and fairly
- Autonomy—the patient's right to making a decision

CAPACITY

Capacity is a person's ability to make a decision based on the information provided. As per the Mental Capacity Act 2005, all patients are presumed to have capacity regardless of age, appearance, disability, beliefs, behavior or treatment decisions against medical advice. Furthermore, capacity is decision-specific and therefore must be assessed on an individual basis.

To be deemed as having capacity, a patient must be able to:

- Understand the information provided
- Retain the information for long enough to make a decision
- Weigh up the information provided and understand the alternatives
- Communicate their decision without being under duress

Where a patient's capacity is called into question, all efforts must be made to ensure:

- There are no impeding factors (for example hard-of-hearing or poor eyesight)
- Involvement of family, friends, Carers or other health professionals involved in their care (GPs, nurses)

For a competent patient who refuses recommended treatment, you must ensure their wishes are respected. All efforts must be made to alleviate their concerns and support them in their decision-making.

DOI: 10.1201/9781003221739-6

In a patient who lacks capacity, determining their best interests should take into account the following considerations:

- Best interests meeting with Next-Of-Kin (NOK), relatives, or lasting power of attorney
- Seeking an Independent Mental Capacity Advocate (IMCA)
- Reviewing any advanced directive and GP records
- Addressing the ceiling of care for the patient and their resuscitation status
- Risk scores of morbidity and mortality related to surgery such as PPOSSUM and NELA scoring for operative morbidity and mortality risk
- Multidisciplinary team meeting (surgical team, anesthetists, nursing staff, other relevant specialties)

For a patient who lacks capacity and does not have family, friends or a legal guardian, doctors must involve an IMCA. The role of an IMCA is to safeguard patients with no family or friends, who cannot make serious medical decisions that may have serious consequences for the patient. They provide support for the patient in the decision-making process and can seek advice from others who know the patient well, such as patient Carers. An IMCA cannot consent on a patient's behalf.

CONFLICT OF OPINION

Where there is a conflict of opinion between the responsible medical team and the family and friends of the patient, advice from the hospital legal department should be sought. If a conclusion cannot be reached, a Court of Protection order may need to be obtained if the decision will result in life-sustaining or withholding treatment.

In an emergency, with no advanced directive available, the consultant responsible should ultimately decide with the involvement of other members of the multidisciplinary team and advice from the hospital's legal team. This decision takes the principle of beneficence which is acting in the patient's best interest.

CONSENT

Consent is an agreement by the patient/advocate for a treatment or procedure. It is an ongoing process, where the patient is given sufficient time to weigh up the information, make a decision and change their mind. Patients should be provided with information early and consent between should not be taken in the anesthetic room. Consent must be informed and valid.

For consent to be informed, there must be:

- A discussion of benefits and risks
- A discussion of "material risks" (what is important to the patient)
- A discussion regarding alternative treatments have been explored
- An interactive discussion, allowing for the patient's and/or advocate's questions and concerns to be addressed

For consent to be valid:

- The patient must have capacity; that is they must be able to understand the information, retain the information for long enough to make a decision, weigh up the risks and benefits, understand the alternative treatment options and communicate their decision.
- The patient must be well-informed (relevant information must be supplied, and all efforts made to ensure that the patient understands the information).
- It must be free from coercion.

For patients who choose not to know the risks, it is advised that you:

- Put the patient at ease
- Address the reasons why and correlate this with the risk of not undergoing the intervention
- Give them time to consider their decision and the opportunity to change their mind at a later date (*Consent is an ongoing process*)

As a prerequisite, you will not be able to proceed unless the patient is fully informed, and this must be explained to the patient.

There are three types of consent:

- Implied: patient undresses for an examination; patient sticks arm out for blood pressure to be taken
- Verbal: simple procedures such as blood taking, catheterization
- Written: operative procedures, fertility treatment

WHO SHOULD SEEK CONSENT

- The clinician who is proposing the treatment/carrying out the treatment or a suitably trained/qualified delegate

WRITTEN CONSENT

For most surgical procedures, written consent is required. You should only seek consent from a patient if you have carried out the procedure yourself or you have received training to consent for the procedure. The following standard consent forms allow for the provision of information and confirmation that a decision has been reached based on this:

- Consent form 1—for adult patients or competent young person (Gillick competent)
- Consent form 2—parental consent for a child or young person
- Consent form 3—for procedures where the patient's consciousness is not impaired, i.e. under local or regional anesthesia
- Consent form 4—for the patient who lacks capacity

For treatment decisions where verbal consent is satisfactory, it is imperative that this is recorded in the patient's notes.

STEPS IN OBTAINING INFORMED CONSENT

1. Consultation with the patient from which the doctor gauges the level of understanding of the patient.
2. Doctor describes the available options including:

   - Diagnosis, prognosis and further investigations that are necessary.
   - Different management options available including the outcome of no treatment. The doctor can recommend a preferred course of action but must not coerce the patient.
   - Details of any necessary investigations/treatments/procedures and their purpose.
   - Details of risks (the serious risks, even if very small, and less serious ones), benefits, side effects.
   - Whether the procedure/investigation is part of a research program.
   - Offer the right to a second opinion.
   - Any treatment which the trust cannot provide (e.g. on the grounds of cost and training) but which may be of greater benefit.
   - Also, inform patient about circumstances where further procedures may be necessary during the primary planned procedure, e.g. blood transfusion.

3. Patient weighs up the risks and benefits and determines whether to accept or refuse the proposed options. Allow patient to express concerns.

MATERIAL RISK—MONTGOMERY TEST

Today, informed consent requires patients to be informed of the material risks of a treatment or procedure. The term material risk refers to any risk a person in the patient's position would attach significance to, regardless of its frequency. Identifying what is important to the patient will require taking a thorough history and an open discussion regarding the treatment or procedure. Following the 2015 court case, 'Montgomery vs Lanarkshire', there was a change in the law concerning a doctors' duty to disclose information including material risks. Before Montgomery, a doctor's duty to inform patients of treatment risks was based on whether they had acted in line with a responsible body of medical opinion, also known as the **Bolam test**. The law now requires a doctor to ensure that the patient is aware of any "**material risks**" involved in any recommended treatment and any reasonable alternative treatments.

- **Bolam test** = a test of whether a doctor has acted in line with a responsible body of evidence
- **Montgomery test** = a test of whether a doctor has provided all material risk to a patient (a risk that a patient will attach significance to)

AN ADULT PATIENT WHO LACKS CAPACITY (NON-COMPETENT ADULT)

You must consult the patient's NOK, family or friends to determine the patient's wishes. However, legally, relatives can only give an advisory role.

Unless the patient had signed an advanced directive, the management decision lies with the clinician who must act in the patient's best interest to prevent harm and deterioration (the doctrine of necessity). If the patient regains capacity, then they must be informed of what has happened.

In situations where there are disagreements within the clinician management team, or between the clinician and relatives, it is important to negotiate. The clinician can consult other experienced colleagues for advice.

A consent form 4 must be completed, and all discussions must be clearly documented in the patient's records.

In an emergency situation, where the patient is unconscious/lacks capacity and you are unable to determine their wishes, time-critical intervention that is life-saving or will prevent serious deterioration can be provided. As per the GMC guidance, this should be the least restrictive option and take into account the patients' future options.

CONSENT IN AN UNDERAGE PATIENT (0–18 YEARS)

All children aged 16–18 years can be assumed to be competent. They can give consent to treatment, investigations and procedures. However, in England, Wales and Northern Ireland, they cannot refuse consent to treatment if it has been given by someone with parental responsibility or by the court.

Only guardians with parental responsibility are entitled to consent on behalf of their children. This is not the case for all parents, for example, unmarried fathers or unmarried same-sex partners. It is important to clarify information regarding parental responsibility where there are doubts. In these situations, involvement of both parents, the local safeguarding and paediatric teams are required.

In emergency situations, the GMC guidance outlines that emergency treatment can be provided without consent to save the life or prevent serious deterioration of a child or young person's health. Suppose the parents or legal guardian do not agree with the intervention. In that case, the responsible health professional has the right to override them and proceed with what is in the best interests of the child or young person.

Children under the age of 16 years can give consent only if they are deemed Gillick competent.

Gillick Competency

Gillick Competence is a term given to a young person under the age of 16 who has sufficient maturity and intelligence to understand, weigh up information provided, and decide regarding treatment based on this. A young person who is deemed to be Gillick competent can consent to a procedure or treatment without the involvement of the parent. The term Gillick Competent originates from the legal case in the

1980s regarding whether contraception could be given to under 16s without parental consent.

Anyone under the age of 16 cannot refuse a treatment that is in their best interests. Refusal by a competent young person can be overruled by those with parental responsibility or the court.

Even if a child is competent, every effort should be made to encourage the child to involve their parents. Parents cannot override consent given by a competent child.

Fraser guidelines relate specifically to contraception.

SUMMARY OF CONSENT IN PATIENTS AS DETERMINED BY AGE

Under the age of 16 years	Between the ages of 16 and 18 years	Over the age of 18 years
Can consent to treatment only if Gillick competent	Assumed to have capacity (unless proven otherwise) and can consent to treatment	Assumed to have capacity (unless proven otherwise) and can consent to treatment
Cannot refuse treatment if it has been given by someone with parental responsibility or by the court	Cannot refuse treatment if it has been given by someone with parental responsibility or by the court	Assumed to have capacity (unless proven otherwise) to decline treatment

CARING FOR PATIENTS WHO REFUSE BLOOD TRANSFUSIONS (JEHOVAH'S WITNESS)

In some clinical scenarios, you may be faced with a patient who refuses or cannot receive a blood transfusion. For surgical procedures with a risk of blood loss, it is important to gain consent regarding the transfusion of blood and blood products as part of the consent process.

Many Jehovah's Witnesses (JW) hold religious beliefs against receiving transfusion of blood or blood products. This is not the case for all patients who are JW, and therefore, treatment decisions should not be presumed. Some patients are happy to receive autologous blood transfusion or specific blood products (red cells, platelets, cryoprecipitate, fresh frozen plasma). Therefore, it is important to have a detailed discussion to determine the patient's views to identify appropriate treatment options.

EMERGENCY MANAGEMENT OF A JW PATIENT

A competent, informed JW patient can refuse treatment with blood products (whole blood, red cells, platelets, plasma and cryoprecipitate) and should sign a "refusal of treatment" document. If the adult is unconscious, check their wallet/bag for an advanced directive or card confirming their status and refusal of blood and blood products. If no advanced directive is found but you believe that he/she may be JW, every effort should be made to get information from previous notes, their GP, family or church. You should contact the hospital liaison committee of JW. This committee was established by the Watchtower Society (the governing body of JW) and help to provide advice and assist in locating doctors with expertise in blood-free alternatives.

In the event that you cannot determine the patient's wishes, you must proceed with the best treatment option available with involvement of the multidisciplinary team. All events will need to be carefully documented in the patient's notes. Consideration for blood-free alternatives must be given if this can achieve similar results to blood transfusion. It is important to liaise with your medical defense union or hospital legal team in the event that the patient (after regaining capacity) or family is not happy with your decision and decides to take action.

EMERGENCY TREATMENT OF JW CHILDREN

Medical and nursing staff are not legally required to obtain consent before providing life-saving treatment to a child against their parents' wishes. However, all efforts must be made to involve the parents or legal guardian. As with adults, consideration for blood-free alternatives must be given if this can achieve similar results to blood transfusion. Ideally, two consultants should document that a blood transfusion is essential to save life and prevent harm. If time permits, approval from the high court should be sought as it can overrule parents' approval and keep them fully informed.

Treatment options if there is adequate consent for the refusal of blood transfusion:

- Ensure the patient is consented for blood loss and the implications of not receiving a blood transfusion
- Involve the hematology team
- Consider tranexamic acid (antifibrinolytic), plasma expanders if actively bleeding
- Employ the use of a cell saver in theater if autologous transfusion (contact theater coordinator early)

DUTY OF CANDOUR

Duty of Candour refers to a doctor's professional obligation to being open and honest with patients when things go wrong. As of 2014, a new legislation was introduced making this a statutory duty.

As part of this, surgeons are expected to:

- Disclose to the patient immediately when a mistake has been made involving their care
- Provide them with detailed information regarding this if known at the time and if there is any information missing
- Answer questions truthfully and fully
- Offer a verbal apology and where required, a written one
- Describe the short and long-term implications of this mistake

- Offer suitable options for resolution of the mistake and support the patient
- Where relevant, explain how this mistake will be prevented from happening again
- Ensure that any discussion is documented carefully in the patient's notes

Details of how to implement this statutory duty are outlined in the Royal College of Surgeon's guidance on Duty of Candour.

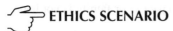 ## ETHICS SCENARIO

The following is a clinical management scenario from a recent interview. There are multiple ethical issues raised, and you will be expected to discuss these as part of your management strategy.

You are asked to organize a day case list for your consultant who is currently in a meeting.

An example of how to approach this scenario:

1. A 30-year-old man listed for a laparoscopic cholecystectomy with a diagnosis of biliary colic. You are informed by the anesthetist that the patient has learning difficulties and is concerned he doesn't have capacity. The patient does not have a Next-Of-Kin.
2. A 20-year-old woman listed for a laparoscopic cholecystectomy with a diagnosis of recent gallstone pancreatitis. A urine dipstick prior to surgery is positive for pregnancy. The patient is unaware of this.
3. A 53-year-old man listed for a laparoscopic Nissen fundoplication for severe reflux disease. The patient has had their operation cancelled twice. He is worried it will happen again and is becoming aggressive.

Breakdown of scenario:

1. The anesthetist has concerns regarding the patient's **capacity** based on the fact that he has a learning disability. As a rule of thumb, all patients are presumed to have capacity regardless of underlying disability. First, you will need to find out more information from the anesthetist. You will need to review all medical records (clinic letters, inpatient notes) prior to reviewing the patient and then review the patient yourself and assess if they have capacity.

   If you determine the patient lacks capacity, they will not be able to undergo the procedure on this list; however, all efforts must be made to find out more about the situation. This patient apparently does not have a NOK. This must be verified by contacting the GP to find out if there are any guardians of responsibility. The consultant should be informed. If you feel upon review with the consultant that a laparoscopic cholecystectomy is in their best interests, prior to discharge, an **IMCA** should be sought to appropriately consent the patient. A **consent form 4** should be signed. This should be ideally completed before the patient is discharged and you should liaise with the waiting-list coordinator to ensure that the patient is relisted. It would be prudent to arrange a follow-up clinic appointment to ensure that the patient is not lost in the system. This should all be discussed with the responsible consultant, and all events should be clearly documented in the patient's notes.

2. In this situation, the patient is unaware that she is pregnant so will need to be informed in the first instance. From a clinical standpoint, surgery in pregnancy requires careful consideration of the stage of pregnancy, risk of harm to the patient and risk of harm to the baby. Operating in the first trimester as a general rule should be avoided unless absolutely necessary. Gallstone pancreatitis has a significant risk for both mother and miscarriage of pregnancy and the risk of recurrence and severity of previous illness needs to be considered.

   Considering she has **capacity** and based on the principle of **autonomy**, she has the right to make the decision and may decide she would like to go ahead with the cholecystectomy in view of her risk of recurrent gallstone pancreatitis. If further workup of the pregnancy is required, this needs to be done as soon as possible, and involvement of the obstetrics and gynecology team is imperative. Ultimately, the patient will not be able to go ahead on the list until the situation is clarified and she has been reviewed by the consultant. It may be prudent to admit the patient for an inpatient cholecystectomy with appropriate monitoring.

3. The gentlemen who is awaiting a Nissen fundoplication is frustrated and concerned about being cancelled again. It is important to address his concerns and try to put him at ease. You will also need to identify why he had cancelations previously—was there a clinical issue, or was it due to logistical issues in the hospital? If this is the case, this needs to be explained to the patient. As per the principle of **Justice**, all patients should be treated fairly and equally. If he feels he has not received this, it is important to address his concerns and offer an apology. Provided there are no anesthetic or preoperative concerns, and he has been appropriately consented, his operation can go ahead, and he can be placed first on the list.

For all three patients, you will need to do the following:

- Inform the consultant in the first instance.
- Hold a theater briefing with the anesthetic team, theater staff, coordinator.
- Ensure the patients are kept informed and if their operation is cancelled, a plan is in place prior to their discharge.
- Ensure all patients who are going ahead with surgery are appropriately consented, have adequate pre-operative bloods, COVID-19 swab if this is during the COVID-19 pandemic and have group and save and cross-match as appropriate.

7 Interview Technique and Tips

PREPARATION IS KEY

The interview is not an exam, but the preparation should be done with the same vigor as for an exam. You have a limited amount of time on the day to convince the interviewers that *you* should be selected for the post, ahead of hundreds of other candidates. The only way to do this in the limited time frame of the interview is to ensure that you know your CV and portfolio well and that your answers are prepared in such a way that would reflect this. This will help you sell yourself better. Lack of preparation could hamper your performance in delivering all of the key points to score the marks on the day. Therefore, there is no substitute for sound preparation.

FAMILIARIZE YOURSELF WITH PERSON SPECIFICATION AND COMPETENCIES EXPECTED

As you go through your CV and portfolio, think of how you meet the person specification and use your portfolio to write down examples. The interviewers in their selection processes will be assessing whether you meet the person specification, so you need to make sure that your answers are themed around this.

WRITE DOWN SOME OF YOUR ANSWERS

The aim of this is not for you to learn paragraphs and recite the person specification verbatims on the day of the interview. It is to help you plan your answers to specific questions. On the day of the interview, nerves can get in the way, and under pressure, you may forget certain points you wanted to mention, or you may end up going off-topic. Writing down your answers ahead of time will help focus the content that you want to deliver on the day. Writing down your answers in bullet point format may be helpful.

PRACTICE YOUR ANSWERS

This is so that your technique and presentation of your answers are as best as possible on the day. This will only come with the practice of delivery of your answers. Practice with another colleague or with seniors and, importantly, ask for feedback.

FOLLOW ALL PRE-INTERVIEW INSTRUCTIONS AND BE PUNCTUAL

The venue and time will usually be provided with enough notice to help you prepare for your travel. Give yourself plenty of time for travel so that you're not running late

DOI: 10.1201/9781003221739-7

as this will make you flustered. Arrive early so that you have extra time to settle and calm your nerves ahead of the interview. Read all instructions carefully and address any queries ahead of the day of the interview.

DRESS FOR SUCCESS

Dress smart and professional to make a positive impression.

BODY LANGUAGE

Sit up straight, do not slouch, do not fidget. Smile and maintain good eye contact as you deliver your answers. Look confident and professional.

DELIVERY OF YOUR ANSWERS

Listen carefully to questions before you begin your answer. Pause and take a moment before you deliver your answer. If you feel nervous at any stage, take a deep breath to help manage any feelings of anxiety. Be truthful and use examples to tie your skills and accomplishments to the person specification. Make sure that you have practiced delivering answers to common questions ahead of the actual interview. Strong answers are specific and succinct.

BUILD RAPPORT WITH THE INTERVIEWER

Introduce yourself, shake hands, smile and be confident. Be polite. Don't interrupt the interviewers. If you do not understand the question, ask the interviewer to repeat it. This is likely to leave a lasting positive impression on the interviewer.

VIDEO INTERVIEWS DURING THE COVID-19 PANDEMIC

The COVID-19 pandemic has changed the way interviews are conducted across many sectors, including medicine. To maintain social distancing and minimize the risk of viral spread, video rather than face-to-face interviews will be conducted. Preparing for a video interview is similar to preparing for a face-to-face interview in that the questions asked and how you conduct yourself will be the same. However, while this format has rapidly gained popularity during the pandemic, it brings its unique challenges that need to be understood. Aside from issues with internet connectivity and delays, some candidates are simply put off by a camera. The key thing to remember is that this is still a real interview, and you will need to prepare for it like you would for a face-to-face interview. Following are a set of tips for preparing for video interviews:

1. Understand the format of the interview and its provider, e.g. Microsoft teams or Skype and ensure that you have downloaded the relevant application. Take time to familiarize yourself with the software. A few days before the

interview, you are advised to conduct trial runs with family or friends to ensure that you have a grasp of it ahead of the interview date.

2. Test the technology to ensure that the picture and sound are clear and make sure that on the day your laptop is fully charged up.

3. Plan your designated space where the interview will take place. Choose a quiet space or room where you will not be disturbed by noise or other people. Ensure that everyone in the house knows that you are starting an interview to not get disturbed. If you have a loud doorbell, make sure that this is disabled for the duration of your interview. If you have small children, they should preferably not be in the house for the duration of your interview.

4. Ensure that the interview space is neat, with good lighting and good internet connectivity. Make sure that your light source is behind the computer, not behind you.

5. Consider using earphones for better sound quality and check this in advance of the interview.

6. Choose a suitable background for your interview. Stick to a plain or blurred background and avoid anything distracting for the interviewers so that the focus will be on you.

7. Disable any software on your computer that might play sounds or notifications.

8. Switch your phone off.

9. Dress smartly. You may be at home, but this is still a job interview, and you want to look professional. You should wear the same smart outfit you would have chosen for a face-to-face meeting with the employer.

10. Use positive body language and ensure that your camera is positioned at eye level. Avoid slumping and fidgeting. Maintain a good posture but sitting up straight, smile and make eye contact. While actual eye contact is not possible by video, you'll want to get as close to that as possible, which means looking at someone's face.

Sometimes, unexpected technical glitches do occur on the day. For example, the sound quality may be suboptimal, and you may not be able to hear the questions very well despite your best preparatory efforts. Make sure you mention this problem right away so that it can be addressed. Don't try to soldier on, as this will hamper your performance. Do practice your video interview skills ahead of time.

Last but not least, this is your opportunity to make a good impression and show what you have to offer. Remember to be confident and show them your best self! Good luck!

Bibliography

1) A Benjamin. (2008). Audit: How to do it in practice. *British Medical Journal*. 31:336 (7655).

2) C Gray. (2005). What is clinical governance? *British Medical Journal*. 330:5254.

3) Doctors Academy. (2021). *MRCS Course* [Online]. Available from: www.courses. doctorsacademy.org.uk [Accessed 19/07/2021].

4) F Myint. (2019). *Kirk's Basic Surgical Techniques*. Seventh Edition. London: Elsevier Ltd.

5) Health Education England. (2019). *2019 ST3 General Surgery and Vascular Surgery: Supplementary Applicant Handbook* [Online]. Available from: www.oriel.nhs.uk/web/ [Accessed 15/07/2020].

6) Health Education England. (2021). *Person Specification 2021: General Surgery— ST3* [Online]. Available from: https://specialtytraining.hee.nhs.uk/portals/1/Content/ Person%20Specifications/General%20Surgery/GENERAL%20SURGERY%20 %E2%80%93%20ST3%202021.pdf [Accessed 19/07/2021].

7) Intercollegiate Surgical Curriculum Programme. (2017). *Core Surgical Training* [Online]. Available from: www.iscp.ac.uk/curriculum/surgical/specialty_year_sylla-bus.aspx?enc=Tlq9NY9MM5ZH/u9+LCxOLA== [Accessed 19/07/21].

8) J Beard & P Gaines (eds.). (2005). *Vascular and Endovascular Surgery—A Companion to Specialist Surgery Practice*. Third edition. London: Saunders Ltd.

9) J Jameson & D Bryden (eds.). (2017). *Care of the Critically Ill Surgical Patient: Student Handbook*. Fourth edition. London: The Royal College of Surgeons of England.

10) J Kurz, A Hague, G Perin & S Balasubramanian. (n.d.). *What Is Critical Appraisal, Why Is It Important and What Can You Do to Develop Your Appraisal Skills?* [Online]. Available from: www.cramsurg.org/blog/criticalappraisal/index.html [Accessed 19/07/2021].

11) National Institute of Clinical Excellence. (2021). *Guidance and Advice List* [Online]. Available from: www.nice.org.uk [Accessed 19/07/2021].

12) OJ Garden (ed.). (2009). *Hepatobiliary and Pancreatic Surgery—A Companion to Specialist Surgery Practice*. Fourth edition. London: Saunders Ltd.

13) P Jonsson & J Bouvy. (2018). Research governance policy. *National Institute for Health and Care Excellence* [Online]. Available from: www.nice.org.uk/Media/Default/About/ what-we-do/science-policy-and-research/research-governance-policy.pdf [Accessed 19/07/2021].

14) R Patel. (2016). How to prepare for the ST3 general surgery application. *British Medical Journal*. 352:i352 [Online]. Available from: www.bmj.com/content/352/bmj.i352 [Accessed 19/07/2021].

15) Royal College of Surgeons of England. (2020). *Interviews for Surgical Posts* [Online]. Available from: www.rcseng.ac.uk/careers-in-surgery/trainees/foundation-and-core-trainees/how-to-get-ahead-in-surgery/interviews-for-surgical-posts/ [Accessed 19/07/2021].

16) S Clark (ed.). (2019). *Colorectal Surgery—Companion to Specialist Surgery Practice*. Sixth edition. London: Elsevier Ltd.

17) SM Griffin & SA Raines (eds.). (2009). *Oeosphagogastric Surgery—Companion to Specialist Surgery Practice*. Fourth edition. London: Saunders Ltd.

18) S Paterson-Brown (ed.). (2014). *Core Topics in General and Emergency Surgery— Companion to Specialist Surgery Practice*. Fifth edition. London: Saunders Ltd.

19) Social Care Institute for Excellence. (2010). *Mental Capacity Act: Information for Doctors about Medical Decisions* [Online]. Available from: www.scie.org.uk/mca/imca/info-for/doctors [Accessed 19/07/2021].

20) The Committee on Trauma. (2018). *ATLS Advanced Trauma Life Support: Student Course Manual*. Tenth edition. Chicago: American College of Surgeons.

21) The General Medical Council. (2021). *Ethical Guidance for Doctors* [Online]. Available from: www.gmc-uk.org/ethical-guidance/ethical-guidance-for-doctors [Accessed 19/07/2021].

22) The General Medical Council. (2021). *Openness and Honesty When Things Go Wrong: The Professional Duty of Candour* [Online]. Available from: www.gmc-uk.org/ethical-guidance/ethical-guidance-for-doctors/candour-openness-and-honesty-when-things-go-wrong [Accessed 19/07/2021].

23) The Royal College of Surgeons of England. (2020). *Caring for Patients Who Refuse Blood* [Online]. Available from: www.rcseng.ac.uk/standards-and-research/standards-and-guidance/good-practice-guides/patients-who-refuse-blood/ [Accessed 19/07/21].

24) The Royal College of Surgeons of England. (2020). *Duty of Candour* [Online]. Available from: www.rcseng.ac.uk/standards-and-research/standards-and-guidance/good-practice-guides/duty-of-candour/ [Accessed 19/07/21].

25) The Royal College of Surgeons of England. (2020). *Good Surgical Practice* [Online]. Available from: www.rcseng.ac.uk/standards-and-research/gsp/ [Accessed 19/07/21].

26) V Taylor. (2012). *Leading for Health and Wellbeing*. Thousand Oaks, CA: SAGE Publications Ltd.

27) W Bennis & B Namus. (1985). *Leaders: The Strategies for Taking Charge*. New York: Harper & Row.

Index

A

abdominal aortic aneurysm (AAA) repair, 20–22, 48–49
abdominal trauma, 29–32, 34–36
abstracts, xix
academic degrees, 5
academic station
    evidence-based medicine, 13–14, 59–60
    overview, xix, 59
acute limb ischemia, 22, 53, 57
Advanced Trauma Life Support (ATLS), 6, 26, 31
American Association of Surgery, 29
American Society of Anesthesiology (ASA), 19
anastomotic dehiscence, 26
appendicectomy, 3
Assessment of Airway, Breathing, Circulation, Disability and Exposure (ABCDE), 18, 19, 21, 22, 23, 24
audit cycle, xix, 10
audits, xix, 4–5, 10–12, 13
automobile collision trauma, 33–36, 52–53
autonomy, 74, 81
awards, 6

B

Basic Surgical Skills, xix
beneficence, 73, 74
bilateral calf pain, 40–42
blind studies, 61
blood transfusions, 78–79
boils, 39–40
Bolam test, 76

C

CAMP framework, 9
capacity, xix, 18, 38–39, 73–74, 75, 77, 78, 80–81
career progression, 1
Care of the Critically Ill Surgical Patient (CCrISP), 6, 18, 20, 22, 23, 24
case-control studies, 60, 61
case report, 60
case series studies, 60
cholecystectomy, 3
chronic obstructive pulmonary disease, 17–18
clinical effectiveness, 13
clinical experience, 60
clinical governance, xix, 13
clinical management station
    clinical scenarios, 46–54, 80–81

overview, xviii, 45
preparation, 45–46
prioritization scenarios, 54–58
clinical scenarios
    clinical management station, 46–54, 80–81
    ethics station, 80–81
    patient in clinic, 36–43
    technical skills station, 69–71
    trauma call, 26–36
    unwell patient in A&E, 18–26
    unwell patient on the ward, 18–26
    unwell patient on the ward scenario, 51–52
clinical skills, 1
clinical station
    clinical scenarios, 18–43
    format, 18–43
    overview, xviii, 17
    preparation, 17–18
cohort study, 60, 61
colorectal cancer, 36–39
communication issues, 54
communication scenarios, 54–58
communication skills, 1, 14–15
comparative studies, 60
competency-based questions, 9
conferences, 4
conflict of opinion, 74
consent, xix, 2, 12, 24, 29, 35, 38, 53, 54, 74–79, 81
consent forms, 5, 29, 53, 75, 77, 79, 81
Consolidated Standards of Reporting Trials (CONSORT), xix, 61
consultants
    unavailability, 50–51, 53–54
    updates, 54–58
control groups, 60–61
control study, 60
Core Skills in Laparoscopic surgery, xix, 6
Core Surgical Training, 1, 6
correlation studies, 60
courses, 6
Court of Protection, 39
Covid-19 pandemic, 7, 16
critical appraisal, 62–63
critical ischemia, 41
cross-sectional studies, 61
curriculum vitae, xviii

D

data collection, 11
decision-making skills, 1

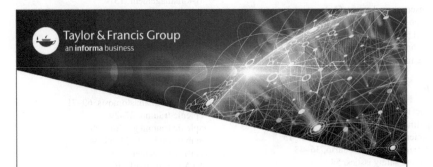